PSYCHIATRY – THEORY, APPLICATIONS AND TREATMENTS

SCHIZOPHRENIA

ADVANCES IN RESEARCH AND FUTURE DIRECTIONS

PSYCHIATRY – THEORY, APPLICATIONS AND TREATMENTS

Additional books and e-books in this series can be found on
Nova's website under the Series tab.

PSYCHIATRY – THEORY, APPLICATIONS AND TREATMENTS

SCHIZOPHRENIA

ADVANCES IN RESEARCH AND FUTURE DIRECTIONS

BOJAN STERENBORG
EDITOR

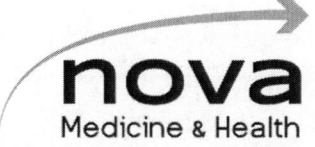

Copyright © 2020 by Nova Science Publishers, Inc.

All rights reserved. No part of this book may be reproduced, stored in a retrieval system or transmitted in any form or by any means: electronic, electrostatic, magnetic, tape, mechanical photocopying, recording or otherwise without the written permission of the Publisher.

We have partnered with Copyright Clearance Center to make it easy for you to obtain permissions to reuse content from this publication. Simply navigate to this publication's page on Nova's website and locate the "Get Permission" button below the title description. This button is linked directly to the title's permission page on copyright.com. Alternatively, you can visit copyright.com and search by title, ISBN, or ISSN.

For further questions about using the service on copyright.com, please contact:
Copyright Clearance Center
Phone: +1-(978) 750-8400   Fax: +1-(978) 750-4470   E-mail: info@copyright.com.

NOTICE TO THE READER

The Publisher has taken reasonable care in the preparation of this book, but makes no expressed or implied warranty of any kind and assumes no responsibility for any errors or omissions. No liability is assumed for incidental or consequential damages in connection with or arising out of information contained in this book. The Publisher shall not be liable for any special, consequential, or **exemplary damages resulting, in whole or in part, from the readers' use of,** or reliance upon, this material. Any parts of this book based on government reports are so indicated and copyright is claimed for those parts to the extent applicable to compilations of such works.

Independent verification should be sought for any data, advice or recommendations contained in this book. In addition, no responsibility is assumed by the Publisher for any injury and/or damage to persons or property arising from any methods, products, instructions, ideas or otherwise contained in this publication.

This publication is designed to provide accurate and authoritative information with regard to the subject matter covered herein. It is sold with the clear understanding that the Publisher is not engaged in rendering legal or any other professional services. If legal or any other expert assistance is required, the services of a competent person should be sought. FROM A DECLARATION OF PARTICIPANTS JOINTLY ADOPTED BY A COMMITTEE OF THE AMERICAN BAR ASSOCIATION AND A COMMITTEE OF PUBLISHERS.

Additional color graphics may be available in the e-book version of this book.

Library of Congress Cataloging-in-Publication Data

Names: Sterenborg, Bojan, editor.
Title: Schizophrenia : advances in research and future directions / [edited by] Bojan Sterenborg. Description: Hauppauge : Nova Science Publishers, [2020] | Series: Psychiatry - theory, applications and treatments | Includes bibliographical references and index. | Summary: "Schizophrenia is a major psychiatric disorder characterized by a disruption in neuropsychological function that usually manifests itself between the age of 10 and 35. Schizophrenia: Advances in Research and Future Directions provides a broad overview of the domains, severity, and course of neuropsychological functioning in schizophrenia patients. Genetic variations and markers can serve as a diagnostic, prognostic and therapeutic tool for the patients. As such, the authors describe and summarize the blood-based biomarkers of schizophrenia from the diagnostic, prognostic and therapeutic points of view. The closing study aims to determine the role of internalized stigma in the presence and severity of fear of negative evaluation in patients with schizophrenia, specifically hypothesizing that a higher perceived discrimination will be the most important predictor"-- Provided by publisher. Identifiers: LCCN 2020025114 (print) | LCCN 2020025115 (ebook) | ISBN 9781536181449 (paperback) | ISBN 9781536181715 (adobe pdf) Subjects: LCSH: Schizophrenia. | Schizophrenia--Research. Classification: LCC RC514 .S33425 2020 (print) | LCC RC514 (ebook) | DDC 616.89/80072--dc23 LC record available at https://lccn.loc.gov/ 2020025114 LC ebook record available at https://lccn.loc.gov/2020025115

Published by Nova Science Publishers, Inc. † New York

CONTENTS

Preface		vii
Chapter 1	Neuropsychological Functioning in Schizophrenia Patients *Behrooz Afshari*	1
Chapter 2	Blood Biomarkers in Schizophrenia: A Focus on Genetics *Javier Gilabert-Juan and Andrzej W. Cwetsch*	75
Chapter 3	The Role of Internalized Stigma in the Fear of Negative Evaluation in Patients with Schizophrenia *Ana Fresán, Rebeca Robles-García, María Yoldi-Negrete, J. Nicolás Martínez-López, Carlos-Alfonso Tovilla-Zárate, Tania Real, Ricardo Saracco-Alvarez and Eduardo Madrigal*	105
Index		123

PREFACE

Schizophrenia is a major psychiatric disorder characterized by a disruption in neuropsychological function that usually manifests itself between the age of 10 and 35. Schizophrenia: Advances in Research and Future Directions provides a broad overview of the domains, severity, and course of neuropsychological functioning in schizophrenia patients.

Genetic variations and markers can serve as a diagnostic, prognostic and therapeutic tool for the patients. As such, the authors describe and summarize the blood-based biomarkers of schizophrenia from the diagnostic, prognostic and therapeutic points of view.

The closing study aims to determine the role of internalized stigma in the presence and severity of fear of negative evaluation in patients with schizophrenia, specifically hypothesizing that a higher perceived discrimination will be the most important predictor.

Chapter 1 - Schizophrenia is a major psychiatric disorder characterized by a disruption in neuropsychological function. The disorder usually manifests itself between the age of 10 and 35, but according to recent researches may already begin during prenatal development. Impairments in a variety of neuropsychological functioning are found in patients with schizophrenia. These impairments affect a wide range of abilities and are often quite severe when compared to standards based on healthy individuals of the same age, education levels, and gender. Although the current knowledge base regarding neuropsychology in the schizophrenia is quite broad, additional research information is accruing. Clinical researches showed broad neuropsychological impairments e.g., executive and cognitive dysfunctions in schizophrenia patients. Many studies have pointed to neuropsychological deficits in Schizophrenia. Higher levels of neuropsychological deficits in schizophrenia patients are associated with frequent hospitalizations, behavioral, emotional, and cognitive responses. Although the mechanism underlying neuropsychological deficits in individuals is unclear, many researchers have pointed to the fundamental effects of genes on brain function and cognitive deficits. These deficits are associated with psychological dysfunctions in areas such as job performance, communication with family members, and life satisfaction. Also, the neuropsychological function is associated with the severity of symptoms in mental disorders. Numerous neuropsychological dysfunctions in schizophrenia have been identified, notably, that executive and cognitive deficits have widespread and significant impacts on the lives, indicating severe problems in controlling and regulating their behaviors. The effects of neuropsychological functioning are so great that we can refer to it as the basis of almost all of the disorders in the DSM-5. The neuropsychological functioning and its evaluation methods are different from the neurological disorders present in DSM-5. The major flaw in the diagnostic criteria for neurological disorders present in the DSM-5 is a misunderstanding of clinical neuroscience assessment, especially neuropsychological functioning. In this chapter, the authors present the neuropsychological aspects of schizophrenia, with emphasis upon the executive and cognitive dysfunctions that are affected. Indeed, the main purpose of this chapter is to provide a broad overview of the domains, severity, and course of neuropsychological functioning in schizophrenia patients.

Chapter 2 - Schizophrenia is a chronic mental disorder characterized by abnormal behavior and a decreased ability to interpret reality. Due to its complexity, during the last few years, many efforts have been made to understand the etiology of the disease and to describe the genetic background responsible for its development. Indeed, numerous studies associated several genes and genetic variants to the pathology. Nevertheless, classical gene studies could not characterize a genetic pool that identifies a specific profile of the patients with schizophrenia. Thus, it is necessary to find genetic expression patterns that allow us to delimit different phenotypes of the disease. Genetic variations and markers can serve as a diagnostic, prognostic and therapeutic tool for the patients. However, limited access to the brain led researchers to look for other, easier to obtain, tissue for marker identification such as peripheral blood. Indeed, many investigations have shown that gene expression in the brain is blood-correlated. Interestingly, genetic markers found in blood include epigenetic changes, alterations in the gene expression and miRNA identification. Here, the authors describe and summarize the blood-based biomarkers of schizophrenia from the diagnostic, prognostic and therapeutic point of view. Finally, the authors will further discuss the future perspectives and the translational aspect of the latest discoveries in the field of schizophrenia research.

Chapter 3 – *Introduction.* Fear is conceived as a normal reaction to threat and is related to a function of survival. However, some people may experience an intense and persistent fear or embarrassment in social situations where they are under the observation or examination of others. This may reflect a core feature of social anxiety, a disorder which interferes with everyday activities. Social anxiety and subthreshold symptoms, defined as an excessive fear of negative evaluation (FNE) from others leading to avoidance of social interactions, is a common comorbid condition among people with schizophrenia, with a deleterious effect on global functioning and quality of life.

Fear of negative evaluation might emerge from several factors, such as biases in cognitive processing, inadequate self-perception in relation to others, and even variables related to the individual's clinical background such as age of onset, delay in specialized treatment and symptom severity. Nevertheless, as its expression is related to the appreciation of others, factors outside the individuals background are necessary to be considered.

Schizophrenia is one of the most stigmatized mental disorders worldwide. The negative public attitudes and beliefs toward the disorder have negative impact on early diagnosis and adequate specialized treatment of the disorder. Also, another consequence may be the internalization of these stigmatizing conceptions, leading to low self-esteem, hopelessness about treatment and recovery.

Some patients may be more susceptible to the criticism and negative attitudes of others toward the disorder they suffer and, eventually, may express symptoms of social anxiety such as fear of negative evaluation as a response to public and internalized stigma.

Therefore, the present study aimed to determine the role of internalized stigma in the presence and severity of fear of negative evaluation in patients with schizophrenia. Specifically, the authors hypothesized that patients with prominent FNE will report more internalized stigma and that a higher perceived discrimination (internalized stigma dimension) will be the most important predictor of prominent FNE in patients with schizophrenia. The authors further hypothesized that groups differences will be observed in symptom severity at the time of the study, with more pronounced negative and affective symptoms in the group of patients with prominent fear of negative evaluation.

Method. Two-hundred and sixty-nine patients with DSM-IV-TR diagnosis of schizophrenia according to the Structured Clinical Interview for DSM-IV Axis I Disorders (SCID-I) were recruited. Symptom severity at the time of the study were rated using the 5-dimensional model of the Positive and Negative Syndrome Scale (PANSS). The King's Internalized Stigma Scale (ISS) was used for the assessment of three main areas of internalized stigma: perceived discrimination, disclosure about mental illness and positive aspects of mental illness. Finally, for the evaluation of fear of negative evaluation, the Brief Fear of Negative Evaluation Scale – Revised (BFNE-II) was used.

The upper quartile (75%) of the BFNE-II total score was used to divide the sample in those patients with prominent FNE and those with absent/mild FNE. Comparative analyses between groups were performed and a multivariate logistic regression analysis was used to determine risk factors associated to prominent FNE in patients with schizophrenia.

Results. Men accounted for 68.4% (n = 184) of the sample with a mean age of 37 years (S.D. = 10.7). Most of the patients were unemployed (72.1, n = 194) and single (98.9%, n = 266). Age of illness onset was reported at

24.2 (S.D. = 7.) years with 56.1% (n = 151) with a history of previous psychiatric hospitalizations. Using the proposed cut-off point 26.4% (n = 71) of the patients were classified in the group of prominent FNE. Demographic features were similar between FNE groups as well as current psychotic symptomatology assessed with the 5-dimensional model of the PANSS ($p > 0.05$). A greater number of patients with prominent FNE reported previous psychiatric hospitalizations (61.1% vs. 42.3%, $p = 0.006$). The three dimensions that comprise internalized stigma and its total score was significantly higher in patients with prominent FNE ($p < 0.01$) and the dimensions of perceived discrimination and positive aspects of mental illness were predictors of prominent FNE inpatients with schizophrenia (OR = 1.0, 95% C.I. = 1.05 - 1.13 and OR = 1.1, 95% C.I. = 1.08 - 1.30 respectively).

Discussion. Internalized stigma has been associated with higher levels of anxiety in patients with schizophrenia. Although the present study did not determine a definite comorbid social anxiety disorder, the authors' results showed that some patients may have a greater predisposition to fear of negative evaluation in the context of internalization of public stigma. Future studies should address the presence and severity of fear of negative evaluation and internalized stigma in patients with schizophrenia and confidently be differentiated from characteristic symptoms of schizophrenia (as positive and negative symptoms). This, in order to provide effective treatment, pharmacologic and therapeutic for both: anxiety symptoms generated by the fear of negative evaluation and the symptoms of schizophrenia; and thus, reduce as far as possible the social deterioration that the patient could present when having both conditions.

In: Schizophrenia
Editor: Bojan Sterenborg
ISBN: 978-1-53618-144-9
© 2020 Nova Science Publishers, Inc.

Chapter 1

NEUROPSYCHOLOGICAL FUNCTIONING IN SCHIZOPHRENIA PATIENTS

*Behrooz Afshari**
Department of clinical psychology,
Kashan University of medical sciences, Kashan, Iran

ABSTRACT

Schizophrenia is a major psychiatric disorder characterized by a disruption in neuropsychological function. The disorder usually manifests itself between the age of 10 and 35, but according to recent researches may already begin during prenatal development (APA, 2013; Kaplan, 2016). Impairments in a variety of neuropsychological functioning are found in patients with schizophrenia. These impairments affect a wide range of abilities and are often quite severe when compared to standards based on healthy individuals of the same age, education levels, and gender. Although the current knowledge base regarding neuropsychology in the schizophrenia is quite broad, additional research information is accruing. Clinical researches showed broad neuropsychological impairments e.g., executive and cognitive dysfunctions in schizophrenia patients (Afshari, Khezrian, & Faghihi, 2019). Many studies have pointed to neuropsychological deficits in Schizophrenia. Higher levels of

---

* Corresponding Author's Email: behrooz.afshari71@gmail.com.

neuropsychological deficits in schizophrenia patients are associated with frequent hospitalizations, behavioral, emotional, and cognitive responses. Although the mechanism underlying neuropsychological deficits in individuals is unclear, many researchers have pointed to the fundamental effects of genes on brain function and cognitive deficits. These deficits are associated with psychological dysfunctions in areas such as job performance, communication with family members, and life satisfaction. Also, the neuropsychological function is associated with the severity of symptoms in mental disorders. Numerous neuropsychological dysfunctions in schizophrenia have been identified, notably, that executive and cognitive deficits have widespread and significant impacts on the lives, indicating severe problems in controlling and regulating their behaviors. The effects of neuropsychological functioning are so great that we can refer to it as the basis of almost all of the disorders in the DSM-5. The neuropsychological functioning and its evaluation methods are different from the neurological disorders present in DSM-5 (Goldstein, Naglieri, Princiotta, & Otero, 2014). The major flaw in the diagnostic criteria for neurological disorders present in the DSM-5 is a misunderstanding of clinical neuroscience assessment, especially neuropsychological functioning. In this chapter, we present the neuropsychological aspects of schizophrenia, with emphasis upon the executive and cognitive dysfunctions that are affected. Indeed, the main purpose of this chapter is to provide a broad overview of the domains, severity, and course of neuropsychological functioning in schizophrenia patients (APA, 2013; Kaplan, 2016).

A History of Neuropsychological Functioning

Although it is necessary to identify the relationship between one's behavior and the brain region affected by changes in the behavior of a person with a specific brain injury, it is important to understand the complex hidden relationships between brain structures before examining such a relationship (Sporns, 2013). Various topics in neuroscience help us get to know these complex relationships.

Neuropsychology is one of the disciplines of neuroscience that offers a special kind of connection between psychology and neuroscience. The specific subject of this science is to study the role of the human brain in the complex forms of mental activity and the search for a neural organization associated with it (Walsh, 1978). In other words, when it comes to the neural mechanisms of the mind's superb activities, we get into the field of neuropsychology. In a sense, neuropsychology is classified into two subsets of clinical and experimental neuroscience. The main distinction between these two subsets is that clinical studies are performed on patients with brain injury, while experimental studies on healthy individuals are reviewed (Denes & Pizzamiglio, 1999). Therefore, the research method differs in two areas of clinical and experimental neuroscience. As a branch of brain research in the last 20 years, neuroscience has been a specialized area of psychology. neuropsychology explains the relationship between the brain and behavior and seeks to understand how the brain acts, for example, what mechanisms are important in thinking, learning, and feeling, how they are initiated, and how they affect human behavior (Heilman & Valenstein, 2003). It is essential to find a correlation between physiological and psychological data because they are often complementary to each other. Research on the structure and function of the brain has produced a vast array of information and knowledge that is of particular importance and importance to the science of psychology. Even though neuroscience, like other fields of science, has advanced substantially in recent years, and neuroscience research that has begun to benefit from hemispheric superiority has led to the emergence of theories of awareness and differences in occupational, cultural, and educational attitudes. There is a long way to go to present a general theory of the relationship between brain activity and psychological processes.

From the combination of the two words neuro and psychology, it can be assumed that the field of neuropsychology is a major focus on the brain and behavior. Therefore, neuropsychology can be defined as the study of the relationship between brain and behavior. The goal of neuropsychology is to understand the relationship and influence of the brain on behavior (Shallice, 1988). Although humans have always been interested in the relationship between brain and behavior, neuroscience is a relatively new and young science. Traditional approaches in neuropsychology have explored the relationship between local damage to a brain region and psychological deficits, but today, neuropsychology is changing methodological and theoretical frameworks to understand how the brain works.

Neuropsychology is a psychology specialty that studies the relationship between brain and behavior. Neuropsychology is a broad discipline with various subdivisions (Caramazza & Coltheart, 2006):

Experimental Neuropsychology: A Study of the Relationship between Brain and Behavior in Non-Humans.

Cognitive neuropsychology: The study of normal cognition in humans.

Behavioral neuropsychology: A combination of behavioral theories and neuropsychological principles.

Clinical Neuropsychology: A Study of the Relationship between Brain and Behavior in Humans.

When a physician requests neuroscience tests, a clinical neuroscientist usually performs the assessment.

In most cases, clinical neuroscientists are trained in both clinical psychology and neuroscience. The primary role of the clinical neuroscientist is to evaluate cognitive function in people with or suspected of having a brain injury. Cognitive functions are those that a person uses to process external and internal received stimuli. They evaluate explicit behaviors and believe that these behaviors provide information about the integrated functioning of the central nervous system (Heilman & Valenstein, 2003).

In most psychological disorders, local damage to the brain is rarely observed. Therefore, the main challenge in this field is to understand abnormal behavior in the form of information processing inefficiency. The inefficient information processing process seems to be more associated with abnormal behaviors than local brain injury (Nuechterlein et al., 2004). Historically, the role of neuroscientists has been to try to differentiate between organic and functional psychoses. The evolution of this field is characterized by the works of Gall, Broca, James, Watson, Lashley, Goldstein, Hallstead, and Luria. Early theories about the relationship between brain and behavior are presented by Gall. According to Gaul's phrenology theory, certain brain areas that are visible in skull bumps are associated with certain behaviors. With the advancement of performance locating, Paul Broca has increased our understanding of language, especially the functions of expressive language (Spreen, Risser, & Edgell, 1995).

Given the principles of psychology in general and the principles of neuroscience in particular, James and Watson ground the need for empirical data in support of cognitive performance theories. He also suggested that we need scientific methods to conduct psychological studies. Lashley and Goldstein's work led to a better understanding of the relationship between brain location and behavior in normal (neurologically) healthy individuals and those with neurological damage. Hallstead and Reitan, through different methods, have demonstrated that evaluating explicit behaviors can be used to accurately identify brain injuries (Donahoe, 1991).

Although current progress in the relationship between neuroanatomical structures and behavior of neuropsychological theory has been rejected, the discovery of neuroanatomical layers of cognitive function remains a major goal of neuropsychology. It is hypothesized that cognitive function depends both on the specific brain location of that function and on the relationships between multiple brain regions.

Over the past decade, the field of neuroscience has led to significant advances in the study of psychological disorders to the extent that neuroscience has now become an indispensable field for the study of psychological disorders. This progress is through the accurate and reliable quantification of the components of cognitive functioning and behavior concerning normal and abnormal mental status, and the development of neuropsychological models of mental disorders (Filskov & Boll, 1981).

Determining the relationship between cognition and the brain is not an easy subject in psychopathology. Many neuropsychology studies of psychological disorders have been conducted on patients taking psychotropic drugs, which may have profound effects on the measurement of cognitive function. Many psychological disorders include mood changes, and so mood and motivation can affect the performance of individuals in neuropsychological tests. In recent years, more attention has been paid to the discovery of specific syndromes and symptoms, not the disease itself. For example, rather than trying to explain schizophrenia as a disease, attempts have been made to neuropsychological explain its specific features, such as paranoid delusions (Frith, 2014).

THE PHYSIOLOGY OF NEUROPSYCHOLOGICAL FUNCTIONING

More than a hundred years have elapsed since Dox and Broca discovered that left hemisphere damage caused speech impediment, but the right hemisphere did not affect speech. Since then, the researchers have acknowledged that the left hemisphere plays a specific role in speech, but speech and speech are not the only left hemisphere specific action because comparisons between the movement of patients with left hemisphere injury and the right hemisphere show that the left hemisphere is involved in movement control. Also, the results of the researchers' experiments emphasize the role of the right hemisphere more than the left hemisphere in analyzing the components of spatial vision (O'Halloran, Kinsella, & Storey, 2012).

In the field of physiology, it is best to focus on the four lobes, the parietal, the temporal, and the frontal, because these four sections require a lot of research.

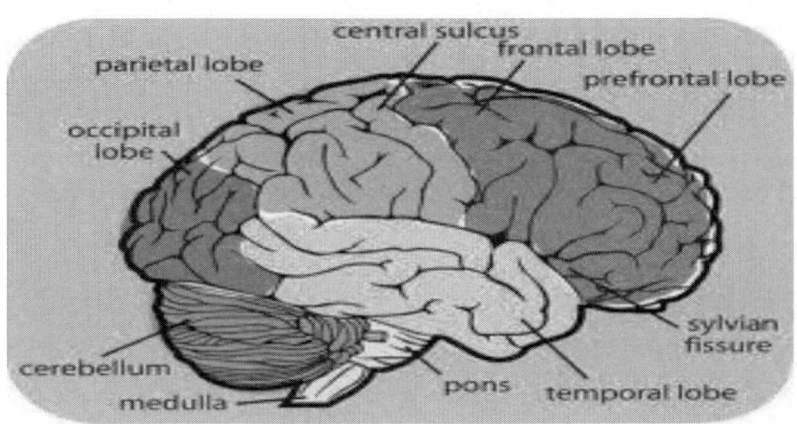

Occipital Lobes

Today, relatively large pieces of information are available on the occipital segment because visual perception and perception are more important to human beings, and therefore more extensive research is being done (Onitsuka et al., 2007). The posterior segment forms the posterior poles of the hemispheres. People with headache damage face visual perception deviations that distinguish objects smaller or larger and lack the necessary visual intensity. In this type of nightmarish, the shape and size of objects change. Also, inhibition of higher cognitive actions leads to the visual agnostic phenomenon that Freud referred to during his career. In such a situation, the patient is not blind and sees the individual properties of objects but cannot fully combine them. It is usually effective in the inability to recognize objects, paintings, and faces in addition to the damage to the occipital segment and temporal lobe injury (Tohid, Faizan, & Faizan, 2015).

Parietal Lobes

The results of the studies show that the frontal and dorsal partial actions are performed independently. One relates more to physical perceptions and perceptions, and the other is to the integration of sensory messages from physical and visual areas (Zhou et al., 2007). The most important piece of parachute action is spatial orientation. In visual-spatial diagnosis, the individual is faced with inhibition in the estimation and orientation of spatial orientation, thus unable to distinguish the direction of the objects towards themselves or toward other objects. It also affects some aspects of spatial memory so that one cannot hold some spatial information in memory (Torrey, 2007). Another of the most important disorders of the parietal fragment is the Grestman's Syndrome, which is characterized by four disorders of written disabilities, inability to identify or name their fingers and others, and failure to recognize left and right. Motor dysfunction is another disorder caused by damage to the parietal part of the brain. The disorder is most commonly seen involuntary movements of the upper body and limbs. In this disorder, the patient is unable to perform or imitate a regular movement task. The most important cases of motor impairment include motor impairment wear and structural motor impairment. In the motor impairment of dressing, the patient cannot wear properly and in structural motor impairment, the individual is unable to organize and fabricate elements (Wingard et al., 2002).

Temporal Lobes

Temporal damage is usually associated with impaired auditory perception, visual perception, classification, memory, emotions, and personality (Goghari, MacDonald III, & Sponheim, 2011).

Hearing Impairment
Bilateral hearing loss may lead to cortical deafness. According to bilateral auditory perception bias, injury in one way does not lead to deafness results from damage in both ears (David, Malmberg, Lewis, Brandt, & Allebeck, 1995).

Visual Perception Disorder
Patients with a right temporal lobe injury have difficulty recognizing faces and remembering them. It also seems that they cannot understand the value of the meaning of visual signs. They also have difficulty drawing and identifying paintings (Heckers, Goff, & Weiss, 2002).

Classification Disorder
The temporal limb plays an important role in organizing sensory messages. Patients with temporal lobe injury find it difficult to classify and organize (Calhoun, Maciejewski, Pearlson, & Kiehl, 2008).

Memory Impairment

The results show that temporal fragments are also important in memory. Some patients develop anterograde amnesia, which means they remember memories of the past but do not recall all the events that happened. Some patients develop amnesia, meaning that they remember all the events after the event but do not recall memories (Pekkonen et al., 2002).

Affective Disorder

Stimulation of the front and middle part of the temporal lobe leads to a feeling of fear, and sometimes stimulation of the lobe also produces this feeling (O. Howes, Jauhar, Brugger, & Pepper, 2018).

Personality Disorder

In people with temporal epilepsy, personality traits such as over-emphasis on the subordinate and mundane issues of everyday life, persistence on personal issues in conversation, self-centeredness, paranoid behavior, overwork in religion, and a tendency to aggressive behavior Observed (O. Howes et al., 2018).

Frontal Lobes

The frontal is usually the location of mental activity and the center of activities that are specific to humans. Important aspects of intelligent behavior are likely related to it. The frontal lobe plays a direct and indirect role in cognitive functions. Some of the disorders that are associated with defects in the frontal lobe include persistence, environmental dependence, and memory disorders (Schoenberg & Scott, 2011). Also, the most important disorders of the frontal lobes can be motor disorders, impaired control and change of behavior, and personality and social behavior disorders. Through the Wisconsin test, it can be shown that the brain flexibility of patients with frontal lobe damage has decreased (Afshari et al., 2019). Patients with frontal lobe injuries also have difficulty in problem-solving processes. Some perceptual deficiencies, such as judgments of body space, also depend on the frontal and frontal cortex.

THE USES OF NEUROPSYCHOLOGICAL FUNCTIONING TASKS

Determining the level of cognitive functioning of the brain is the task of cognitive assessment, which can be performed in various cognitive areas such as reasoning, decision making, learning, memory, and attention, intelligence, and language skills. Cognitive assessment is performed to determine the level of cognitive functioning of the brain in which the individual is asked to complete a set of tasks that require cognitive skills. This assessment can be done in various cognitive areas such as reasoning, decision making, learning, memory, attention, intelligence, and language skills. In this regard, one of the methods of cognitive assessment is the use of neuropsychological tests. It is necessary to know that having the most used tests for assessing cognitive abilities and deficiencies is the need of the world today (John, 2016).

The creation of neurological scales allows for a reliable and valid evaluation of treatment efficacy. The role of clinical neuroscience is to clarify the effects of brain injury on behavior. To this end, clinical neuroscientists measure patient cognitive performance through behavioral tests. The two main approaches in the neuropsychological assessment are quantitative and qualitative. The quantitative approach uses standard scales to measure individuals' cognitive performance compared to what is statistically normal. In the qualitative approach, however, an in-depth analysis is performed by standard scales to find indications of disease index. Although the two approaches have developed independently of each other, current approaches use aspects of both approaches.

Neuroscientists currently use not only these two approaches but also other multidimensional approaches. For example, to measure verbal memory, patients may be asked to keep a list of words. However, this approach is very simple because verbal memory is not just about memorizing words and is more complex; therefore, a full evaluation of verbal memory involves memorizing a list of words, binary words, sentences, short stories, instant recall, delayed recall, And identifying paradigms. Such assessment provides sufficient data to fully analyze specific deficiencies in cognitive abilities and provides the basis for identifying common processes and delineating finer distinctions between abilities and injuries.

Neuroscientists use standardized tests to evaluate people that measure different aspects of psychological functioning. The history of this testing tradition goes back to the early 20th century when French psychologist Alfred Binet began measuring children with brain damage. Tests such as the Alfred Binet test are usually the beginning of the rational assessment, but they also form the basis of psychosocial measurement (Teive, Teive, Dallabrida, & Gutierrez, 2017). Many of the disorders we nowadays diagnose with psychiatric neurological techniques have been identified in binary times. These include dysfunction, dysfunction, perception of distress, and memory deficits.

In 1935, Hallstead founded the Neuroscience Laboratory at the University of Chicago. His main role was to observe people with brain damage. Based on his observations, he identified the behavioral characteristics that should be measured in the neuropsychological testing of patients. The Holstead approach was to use the test set, i.e., to use several different tests that complement each other in measuring the basic categories of psychological function. Ritan made changes to the Hallstead test suite and added a few more tests, such as the Wechsler Intelligence Scale and the Minnesota Multifaceted Personality Meter. The Holsteid-Ritan approach is currently the most widely used test set in neuropsychological assessment. This test is suitable for persons 15 years of age or older. The validity of this set of tests is in separating mentally ill patients whose brains have been damaged by healthy individuals. It is also good for diagnosing lateralization and positioning of brain damage but is poor in separating brain injury from severe mental disorders such as schizophrenia (DeBoskey, 1982; Morlett Paredes et al., 2020).

Another approach was one that emphasized the integrity of the brain rather than the specificity of its regions. This approach was founded by Alexander Luria. Loria's theory was that the brain has three functional systems: 1) the brainstem which regulates the general state or state of awakening; 2) the system that sits in the back of the cerebral cortex and receives information from the outside world and processes it And 3) a system primarily located in the front of the brain that plans, regulates, and executes mental operations. Thus, like other generalists, Loria believed that the brain worked partially, but insisted that we should see how different brain regions work together (Fix, Rougier, & Alexandre, 2007).

Neuropsychologists have been examining the brain function of patients with schizophrenia. Early studies, most of which used the exponential stimulus method, were likely to have schizophrenia due to over-activity of the left hemisphere (Gur, 1978). Current studies also point to the important role of the left hemisphere. The frontal cortex of people with schizophrenia has structural (Sapara et al., 2007) and functional (Harrison et al., 2006) abnormalities. Some studies show that the left frontal area of schizophrenia patients has abnormalities, and the Wisconsin Card Sorting Test shows that the area is not active at the time of the test. Many researchers believe that forehead areas, especially in the left hemisphere, are one of the key features of the brain function of schizophrenia. These results are similar to some observations on schizophrenia symptoms. Many people with schizophrenia show negative symptoms or diminished natural functioning, such as emotional decline, lack of energy, and lack of communication with others. The same symptoms are present in some patients whose affected forehead areas are affected. In patients with schizophrenia, there are also positive symptoms, such as delusions, hallucinations, and strange verbal features. These symptoms are also seen in some areas of the left hemisphere.

Neuropsychological tests are specifically designed tasks used to measure a psychological function known to be linked to a particular brain structure or pathway. They usually involve the systematic administration of clearly defined procedures in a formal environment. Neuropsychological tests are typically administered to a single person working with an examiner in a quiet office environment, free from distractions. As such, it can be argued that neuropsychological tests at times offer an estimate of a person's peak level of cognitive performance. Neuropsychological tests are a core component of the process of conducting a neuropsychological assessment.

In this section, we will mention ten of the most commonly used neuroscience tests used to evaluate schizophrenia patients.

1. Adult Wechsler Intelligence Test

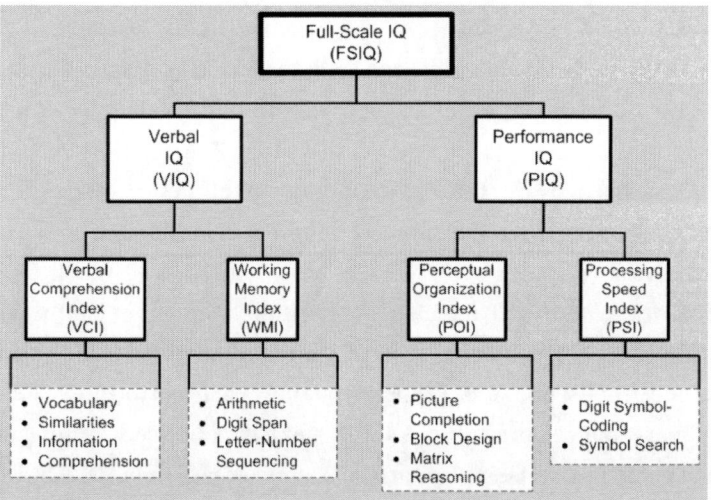

The Wechsler Adult Intelligence Scale contains 4 sub-tests. Of the 3 sub-tests, 2 are verbal and 2 are practical. The Wechsler Intelligence Scale for Children also includes 4 sub-tests, but the important difference between this scale and the Adult Intelligence Scale is that there are two optional sub-tests, called mazes and symbols sub-tests. It reaches 3 sub-tests (Kaufman, Flanagan, Alfonso, & Mascolo, 2006).

The existence of several prominent features, including the ability to measure different domains of IQ and the applicability of subjects of different ages, has made the use of these scales to measure intelligence widely (Littell, 1960).

In his definition of intelligence, Wexler defines it as a general concept that defines one's abilities to perform purposeful activities, rational thinking, and dealing effectively with the environment. Wechsler also does not see the phenomenon of intelligence as a single factor and believes that the state of intelligence can exist in various forms, such as the state of practical, verbal, social, and abstract intelligence. According to Wechsler's definition of the phenomenon of intelligence, he considers it to be a combination of multiple abilities, so he subjected various sub-tests to each of these abilities to measure each of these abilities. (Wechsler, 2012).

Wechsler considers the measurement of children's intelligence to be an effective predictor of children's future behaviors. In his view, the implementation of different IQs can predict many variables such as academic achievement and job success. On the other hand, according to Wechsler, the implementation of IQs can provide valuable information about the strengths and weaknesses of the subject. An important point that Wechsler emphasizes is that by applying intelligence scales one can measure the performance of subjects in different domains and compare them with those of their peers. Wexler also believes that when the test is performed, the tester will have the opportunity to obtain comprehensive information about the individual and individual methods of the test subjects, and finally that Wexler believes that when performing the test IQ can test personal characteristics The subject obtained comprehensive information such as self-esteem, anxiety, and social skills (McCrimmon & Smith, 2013).

Wechsler Intelligence Scales are in a good position in terms of criteria for psychometric evaluation and they are of high standard, validity, and reliability.

Wechsler intelligence scales, like other intelligence scales, have advantages and disadvantages. One of the benefits of these IQs is that the pattern of response to sub-tests of these scales can identify the strengths and weaknesses of the subjects. For example, when sub-test scores are high with a cube and sub-test interpolation, China can be interpreted as having strong perceptual organizing power, or when the subject achieves relatively high scores in the sub-tests of calculating and extrapolating figures. It can be said that he is likely to have a strong short-term memory and not simply distract from doing various tasks. Another advantage of the Wechsler Intelligence Scale is that these scales help measure some of the personality traits of the subjects. For example, a subject who scores low on extracurricular, computational, and digit symbol tests may be predicted to be anxious and less able to concentrate (Jasinski, Berry, Shandera, Clark, & Neuropsychology, 2011). The same can be said about the subject who scores high on the test of comprehension and adjustment of images.

In contrast to the merits of implementing Wechsler intelligence scales, there are some disadvantages to these scales, for example. Intelligence above 1) cannot be measured correctly (Lopez, Stahl, & Tchanturia, 2010).

When performing Wechsler Intelligence Scales, some errors made by the examiner can lead to errors in determining the subject's IQ. Examining the skill of the examiner in performing this test can eliminate many of these errors Some of the common mistakes that Wechsler Intelligence Scale testers make when implementing these scales include: failure to record responses provided by Subject, asking test questions from the test in an inappropriate manner, giving less or more marks to the subject than stated in the test guide, wrong in converting raw scores to standard scores, wrong in calculating the sum of raw scores, and inaccurate (Watkins, 2006).

When the Wechsler Intelligence Scale is completed, the test begins. By finishing the scoring and converting the raw test score to the benchmark score, three types of IQ are obtained under the heading IQ, Verbal IQ, and IQ. Overall IQ is more important than the fact that this type of IQ largely determines the total cognitive power of the subject. Another important aspect of IQ is the high validity and reliability of this type of IQ compared to verbal and practical IQ. Verbal IQ consists of the sum of scores obtained from verbal sub-tests (such as vocabulary tests, parallels, and general information tests), and practical IQ scores from the sum of scores obtained from performing practical sub-tests (such as sub-tests). Composition of parts, design with cubes, and arrangement of images). In general, by examining verbal IQ and practical IQ, the examiner can obtain an estimate of the subjects' perceptual ability to organize. When examining the verbal and practical modality of IQ, the examiner should consider the difference between these two types of IQ. The significant difference between verbal IQ and practical IQ (i.e., scores of 1 to 2) can be attributed to the possibility of minor abnormalities in the functions of the right or left brain hemispheres. If the difference reaches a score of 2 or more, one can judge with greater certainty the possibility of the above abnormality. Wechsler argues that when the score of verbal IQ is much higher than that of practical IQ, small abnormalities in right hemisphere functions can be predicted, and vice versa when practical IQ is much greater than verbal IQ. Small abnormalities in the functions of the left hemisphere of the brain can be predicted (Kaufman et al., 2006).

The main purpose of IQ tests, including the Wechsler Intelligence Scale, is to measure the IQ of the subjects and determine their level or class of IQ. At Wechsler Intelligence Scales, when a person has an IQ of 1 or more, his or her intelligence level is at a very high intelligence level, when the subject's IQ is between 1 and 2, his or her intelligence level is at a high intelligence level, Gaining 110-119 puts the subject's intelligence level above average, a score of 1 to 2 indicates that the subject's level of intelligence is at a medium level when the subject's IQ is above average. Between 1 and 2 indicates that the subject's intelligence level is below average, gaining intelligence; puts the subject's level of intelligence at the borderline level, and gaining intelligence 69 and below places the subject's level of intelligence on the level of subjective intelligence (Watkins, 2006).

Wechsler Intelligence Scale Subtests are

A. Verbal Subtests: General Information Subtest, Digit or Numerical Subtest, Vocabulary Subtest, Mathematics Subtest, Understanding Subtest, Similarities Subtest.
B. Practical Scales: Image Completion Sub-Test, Image Adjustment Sub-Test, Cube Design Sub-Test, Component Testing, and Digit Symbol Test.

2. Stanford Binet Intelligence Test

The Stanford-Binet test was built based on the Alfred Binet and Theodor Simon test. The Binet-Simon Intelligence Test was developed based on two principles: "definition of age" and "concept of general mental abilities". According to the first principle, Binet believed that children's overall mental abilities grow with age. Therefore, the test questions were designed to fit each individual's level of ability. To do this, questions that were answered by between 5% and 5% of people of a particular age group, but younger children less than 2% and older children more than 5%, Selected for the age group. Binet, based on the second principle, focused on measuring intelligence or general mental abilities and did not define and measure the factors that constitute intelligence. Therefore, any question that was correlated with overall ability was included in the test content, and any question that was not correlated with overall ability was excluded. The test, built on the above two principles, consisted of four questions, which were graded by age scale. Then the child's level of intelligence and readiness to use educational facilities were judged by comparing the child's intellectual age and age (Bain & Allin, 2005).

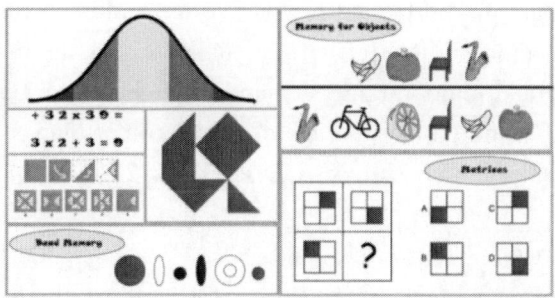

American psychologist Terman translated it into English in nine tests and then standardized it for American children with the help of the Stanford University of California. In this study, Therman retained Binet's principles in making the test but expanded the test content in terms of several questions and age range. For the first time, Therman introduced the concept of IQ based on the formula "IQ = intellectual age divided by age ×

1". This test, which Therman called the Stamford-Binet test, was revised and published once every year, once again in year 2 and its most recent form (Bain & Allin, 2005).

Method of Execution and Grading of the Test

The tester identifies the starting point for the test and the questions, depending on the age, educational background, records, and behavior of the test subject. In the case of normal children and those who appear to be natural intelligence, it is best to begin the experiment with children under one year of age. For example, in the case of a 5-year-old normal child, the test may begin with a 6-year-old child's test questions. If the test determines that the starting point for the test has been selected above the appropriate level, the tester should immediately return to the lower age questions. However, the starting point for asking questions should always be the age at which the subject can answer the questions with minimal effort. Asking questions continues as long as the subject cannot answer any of the questions of one age. At the end of the experiment, the subject's rational age is calculated by considering the age of the starting point and the sum of the points he or she has earned. Refer to the test norm table to determine the intelligence of each individual. The rational table shows the age by month and the horizontal row above the table and time by year in the vertical column to the left of the table. From the intersection of intellectual age and temporal age, deviant intelligence can be found in the table. It should be noted that the age of adults (older than 5 years) at any age is 2 years (Grondhuis, Mulick, & Disabilities, 2013).

Stanford - Binet New Test Form

The fourth revised form of the Stanford-Binet test, the newest form of the test, was developed by Thunderik and Hagen in Year 2. This test has advantages over previous forms of testing. First, the choice of test content and its arrangement is based on a clearer theory of intelligence. Second, in the previous forms of the test, most of the questions were non-verbal, while the new form of the verbal tests was approved. The third advantage is that the test method is such that the content of the test can be quickly and easily matched to the test features. In general, the new form has attempted to address its weaknesses by preserving the positive aspects of the previous test form. In previous forms of the Stanford-Binet test, the subject's intelligence was calculated by age and time. In the new test, the term intellectual age has been removed, and the term "age standard score" is used instead of intelligence. The age criterion score can be determined by comparing the performance of the subject in each sub-test with that of the peer group. The mean score of the age criterion is statistically identical to the concept of intelligence. Because the age standard score is a score where the mean is 100 and the standard deviation is (Roid & Pomplun, 2012).

3. Wechsler Memory Test

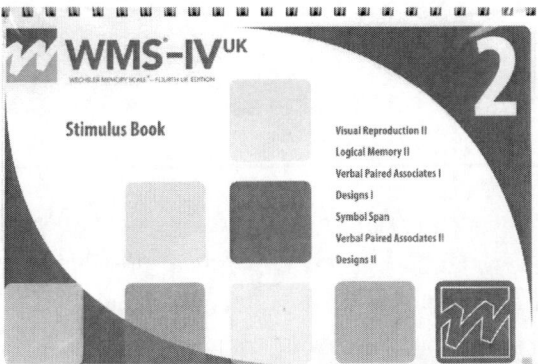

The Wechsler Memory Test, which is used as an objective measure to evaluate memory, has been the result of years of research on and memory of simple, high-frequency memory and provides information to distinguish between functional and functional memory disorders. Wechsler Memory Scale (Form A) consists of 7 sub-tests: 1- Personal awareness of everyday and personal issues 2- Knowledge of time and location 3- Subjective control 4- Logical memory 5- Repeat forward Figures 6- Memory Vision and learning are evocative (Langeluddecke & Lucas, 2003).

The total memory score is obtained from the sum of the subscales of the subjects. According to the standard US standardized test form; we can add to these raw scores a modified fixed score given in Table 2 for different age groups, which yields the sum of these two "rated scores" of cholera. Refer to Table 3 to obtain the memory gain (MQ) equivalent to the scores scored (Kent, 2020).

4. Verbal Fluency Test (VFT)

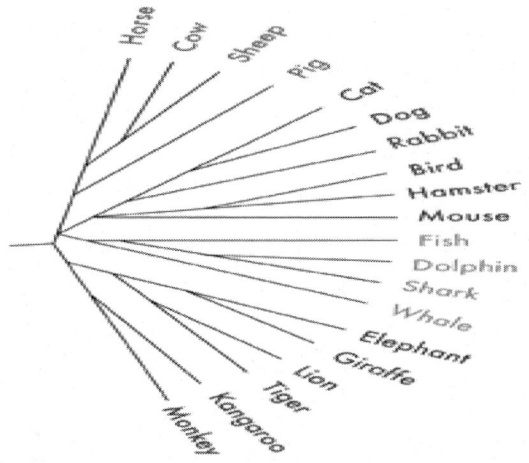

Verbal fluency tests are a kind of psychological test in which participants have to produce as many words as possible from a category in a given time (usually 60 seconds). This category can be semantic, including objects such as animals or fruits, or phonemic, including words beginning with a specified letter, such as *p*, for example. The semantic fluency test is sometimes described as the category fluency test or simply as "free listing". The controlled oral word association test is the most employed phonetic variant. Although the most common performance measure is the total number of words, other analyses such as some repetitions, number, and length of clusters of words from the same semantic or phonetic subcategory, or some switches to other categories can be carried out (Chou et al., 2018).

The verbal fluency test is a short test of verbal functioning. It typically consists of two tasks: category fluency (sometimes called semantic fluency) and letter fluency (sometimes called phonemic fluency). In the standard versions of the tasks, participants are given 1 min to produce as many unique words as possible within a semantic category (category fluency) or starting with a given letter (letter fluency). The participant's score in each task is the number of unique correct words (Ono et al., 2017).

Verbal fluency tasks are often included in neuropsychological assessment, clinical practice, and research.

5. Trial Making Test

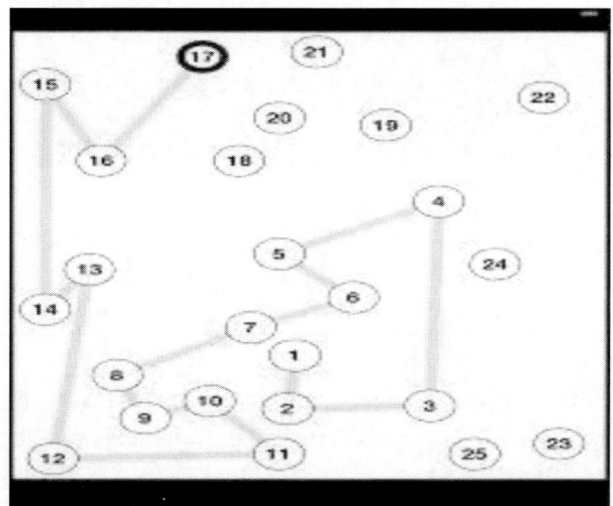

The trail making test (TMT) is a neuropsychological paper-form test that was initially developed by the US army during the Second World War to evaluate overall performance in recruits. During the late'40s and early'50s, two of its creators, Armitage and Reitan, then transposed its application to assess brain injury in patients following stroke. Its ability to assess fitness to drive was first tested in 1992 for patients with closed brain injury and older drivers the following year. Since then, studies have shown the TMT to be one of the best performing paper-and-pencil–based neuropsychological tests in predicting driving difficulties (Kaswan, Thompson, Adler, & Hirst, 2019).

The first part of the TMT measures the time participants need to connect 25 numbered circles in ascending order (part A). In the second part

(B), 13 numbers and 12 letters have to be alternately connected in their numerical and alphabetical order. Participants were notified of errors immediately and required to correct them without assistance with the clock running (Fellows, Dahmen, Cook, & Schmitter-Edgecombe, 2017).

6. Simple Reaction Time (SRT)

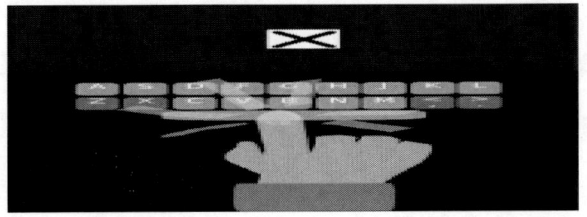

The Simple Reaction Time (RT) Task measures the basic cognitive processes of perception and response execution. The task requires that participants make one specific response (e.g., a spacebar press) whenever any stimulus (e.g., a shape) appears on the screen. Typically, there is only one stimulus that repeats throughout the experiment. This straightforward task engages certain basic processes, such as perception and response execution, without requiring more complicated processes such as attention focusing (i.e., resisting distraction) or response inhibition (i.e., stopping a motor action). The main dependent measure is the speed of responding (Ghisletta, Renaud, Fagot, Lecerf, & De Ribaupierre, 2018; Willoughby, Hong, Hudson, & Wylie, 2020).

7. Selective Attention

Attention is a cognitive process, or brain function that has as its main objective to allocate the cognitive processing towards a stimulus, let it be visual, auditory, or related to some other sense. That is, attention defines which information is most relevant among the various sensory inputs that occur at the same time as the stimulus.

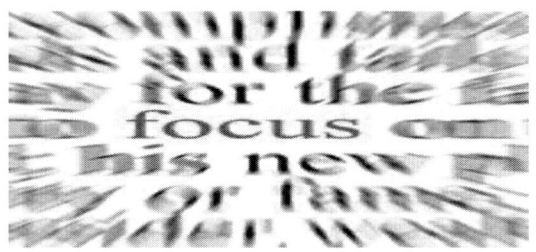

We can define four types of attention, which are: sustained, selective, alternated, and divided.

Selective attention subtype in which we can select, from various factors and characteristics of a stimulus, focus on only one factor of interest. This process occurs concomitantly with the filtering of non-focused parts of the stimulus. In other words, selective attention allows us to select the stimulus that we want to pay attention to (Moray, 2017).

8. Wisconsin Card Sorting Task

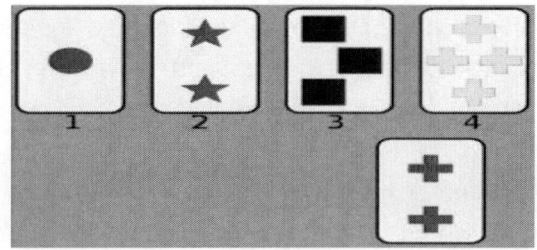

The Wisconsin Card Matching Task is used to measure abstract reasoning, conceptualization, and repetitive response in people ages 6.5 to 89. In this assignment, the patient is asked which cards are presented to him based on Classify one of the three principles of class membership. The scales obtained from this test are as follows: Classifications performed repetitive responses, repeated errors, non-repetitive errors, failure to retain memory, and learning adequacy (Rhodes & aging, 2004).

This test is considered one of the most sensitive tests for the frontal cortex and lateral dorsal cortex. Lazac reported the validity of this test for assessing cognitive deficits following brain injury above 0.86. The reliability of this test was also reported based on the coefficients of agreement of the evaluators in the Sprain and Strauss study of 0.83 (Tchanturia et al., 2012).

How to Run the Wisconsin Test

The test consisted of 64 cards with one of four symbols in the form of red triangles, green stars, yellow crosses and blue circles, and no duplicate or duplicate characters. The task of the tester is to draw cards based on the inference of the pattern used by the tester. This pattern consists of a red triangle, two green stars, three yellow crosses, and four blue circles. The principle of sorting and inserting cards is in the order of color, shape, and number of symbols that the tester considers without the tester's knowledge. When the subject can sort the ten cards consecutively by color, the tester changes the criterion, and the tester must understand this change by saying the tester is "right" and "not right" and finds the new principle.

The test goes on until the subject replaces ten cards for six times or spontaneously reports on the underlying principle, for example, saying "you are constantly changing the principle." I usually stop the test after the 30 to 40 cards are incorrectly inserted and the subject appears to be reluctant to understand the task (Head, Kennedy, Rodrigue, & Raz, 2009).

Wisconsin Test Scoring

The test can be scored in several ways. The most common method of scoring is to record the number of classes achieved and error incompleteness. The obtained classes are referred to as the number of correct periods or in other words ten consecutive correct placements, which range from zero to six in which the test normally stops. There are times when the subject continues to classify following the previous successful principle and also when he persists in the first series in the classification based on an initial false conjecture. The error of persistence is useful and useful for documenting concept formation, benefiting from perceptual correction, and flexibility. Specific errors include errors other than synchronization errors (Parker et al., 2018).

9. London Tower Test

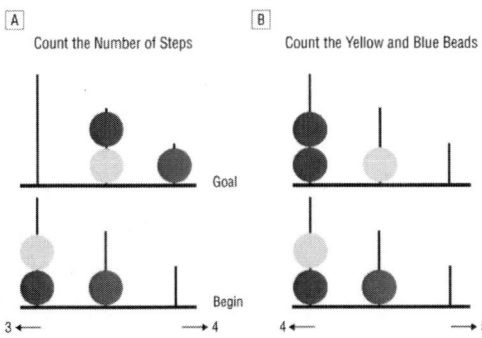

The Tower of London Test was designed by Shallis in 1982 to evaluate the executive function, particularly the detection of planning deficits and impaired ability to solve patients with frontal lobe lesions. The main form of the test performed by Shalis was two boards, each with three bars of varying lengths and three beads. In the Shalis study, patients and controls were asked to move the vertebrae on the workspace to conform to a predetermined pattern. According to Shalis, the ability to solve the problem was determined by the number of additional movements (errors) of the subject compared to the minimum movements required to fit the model. In other words, the greater the number of extra movements a subject had, the less capable of solving the problem is. Shalis concluded that those with lesions in the anterior left frontal lobe were more error-prone than the control group and spent more time (especially at design time before starting) on model alignment. After Shalis, the researchers applied different test forms with more rods and beads without limiting the length of the rod and devised different criteria for scoring and diagnosis. On the other hand, there have also been some critique studies of the validity of the test and factors affecting the ability to solve the problem (such as age, fluid intelligence, etc.) that affect the results of the test. Some studies have demonstrated the successful use of this test to measure planning ability in patients with Alzheimer's, schizophrenia, and attention deficit hyperactivity disorder. There are different computer versions for this test (Boghi et al., 2006; Chang et al., 2011).

Test Tools

There are three main components to this test: boards, bars, and beads. Problem-solving is a skill needed by people of all ages to achieve goals and complete tasks. Cognitive borrowing that has engulfed the minds of cognitive psychologists and neuroscientists for many years. Shalis developed the Tower of London (TOL) in 1982 to measure planning and problem-solving skills in patients with frontal lobe disorders. Patients and controls were faced with a situation that had to be achieved by moving the grains from the current state to the target state and patterns. In Shalissi's study, the power of problem-solving was equal to the number of moves an individual had to make to reach the target status (Phillips, 1999). The higher the number of movements, the less able the person is to solve the problem. According to Shalis, people with injuries in the left anterior region have more errors and more time to plan.

The results of other focused research support Shalice's findings and all suggest that trauma to the peri-frontal region is associated with a defect in problem-solving ability. This test has been widely performed on normal people and people with various disorders such as autism, hyperactivity, dementia, schizophrenia, and research has shown that the result is different in normal and clinical populations (Van Den Heuvel et al., 2003).

Various versions have been produced to accurately measure the problem-solving ability of populations with disabilities with different disabilities. Some computer labs and some versions of bars and actual screens have used that people can do with proper physical conditions. The number of problem-solving moves in different researches with different individuals varied from two to eight. Different studies have also measured different aspects of problem-solving and different criteria. Some count as a measure of problem-solving ability, while others as a measure of problem-solving ability as a whole. And they also have some thinking time before doing the first move. All of these criteria must be considered when interpreting and interpreting the results (Köstering et al., 2015).

10. Continuous Performance Task (CPT)

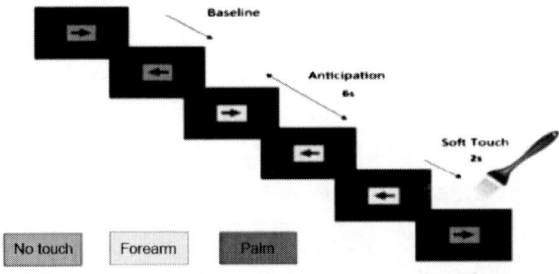

The continuous performance test (CPT) is any of several kinds of neuropsychological test that measures a person's sustained and selective attention. Sustained attention is the ability to maintain a consistent focus on some continuous activity or stimuli, and is associated with impulsivity. Selective attention is the ability to focus on relevant stimuli and ignore competing stimuli. This skill is associated with distractibility (Cope & Young, 2017).

There is a variety of CPT; the more commonly used is the Integrated Visual and Auditory CPT (IVA-2), Test of Variables of Attention (T.O.V.A.), and the Conner's' CPT-III. These attention tests are often used as part of a battery of tests to understand a person's 'executive functioning' or their capacity to sort and manage information. They may also be used specifically to support or to help rule out a diagnosis of Attention Deficit Disorder. Also, there are some CPTs, such as QbTest and Quotient that combine attention and impulsivity measures with motion tracking analysis. These types of CPTs can assist health professionals with objective information regarding the three core symptoms of ADHD: hyperactivity, inattention, and impulsivity (Epstein et al., 2003).

NEUROPSYCHOLOGICAL FUNCTIONING IN MENTAL DISORDERS

Psychologists have long been interested in investigating the cause of mental disorders for many years, and these studies have played an important role in early attempts to classify mental disorders. Neuropsychologists' research has helped to clarify and understand mental disorders. These studies have also expanded our knowledge of childhood to adulthood. We will mention here some of the disorders that have been the subject of most neuroscience research.

Neuropsychologists, who have systematically proven that brain damage can have emotional effects, have also studied the neuropsychology of depression. For example, people whose right hemisphere is damaged usually do not get upset or even care about their mental disorder or hospitalization. This indifference and happiness are usually accompanied by a deficiency or lack of awareness of their defects. But people whose left hemisphere is damaged usually cause a catastrophe, which means they are crying, desperate, and other symptoms of depression. Many studies show that most people become depressed after their left hemisphere is damaged. Studies have also shown that the closer the injury is to the front of the left hemisphere, the greater the likelihood of depression. Also, the activity of the left hemisphere of those with depression is less than that of the right hemisphere. This difference in brain activity is more pronounced in the frontal regions, and this indicates the importance of these regions in producing these emotional states. These neuropsychological findings not only help to understand depression but also help diagnose and treat depression after brain injury. For example, we should consider the possibility that patients with brain damage can be depressed in addition to having difficulty understanding language and speech. This is why neuroscientists ask a person and his or her family members whether sleep and nutrition are normal and whether or not they expect to improve (Groves et al., 2015; Porter, Bourke, Gallagher, & Psychiatry, 2007).

Due to the interest of neuroscientists in their cognitive and cognitive abilities, many are researching their learning, assessment, and treatment disabilities. Much of the work of neuroscientists has been on the role of behavioral, environmental, social, and biological factors in learning disabilities. For example, research by neuroscientists suggests that dyslexia or impaired reading ability is usually linked to left hemisphere malignancy. Studies by brain imaging have also shown that children's reading ability is correlated with left hemispheric neural pathways. Neuropsychologists' assessments can clarify some of the problems in the workings of the left hemisphere and help formulate restorative strategies. Children with school-based attention problems (such as ADHD), memory, or language problems, and social and emotional problems (such as depression and anxiety) are usually referred to as neuroscientists. Discuss and discuss with parents and teachers the best way to help the child (Pauli-Pott & Becker, 2011; H. E. Schneider, Lam, & Mahone, 2016).

Another type of learning disability is a defect in spatial visual and motor skills that is related to the right hemisphere. Children with non-verbal learning disabilities usually have difficulty in non-verbal tasks such as tying shoes, dressing, eating, and adjusting their time. These defects can make it difficult for the child to discover the environment and gain experience. A key point for people who experience the disorder is that they have age-appropriate verbal skills, such as speaking ability and decoding reading ability. But they have weaknesses in social, spatial, visual, and motor skills. Neuroscientists, like other learning disabilities, also design restorative programs related to nonverbal learning disabilities and encourage parents and teachers to work with children on these skills (Wong, 2011).

Another disorder that has received much research in the field of neuroscience is Alzheimer's disease. Many families have a grandparent nursing experience that was active and meticulous some years ago, but now her mental abilities are greatly reduced and she cannot take care of herself. The problem usually starts with mild distractions. Grandfather lost his belongings or asked a question several times. Shortly afterward, Grandfather was no longer able to pursue complicated discussions or formerly simple leisure activities were now challenging him. The early family has attributed these changes to her exhaustion or age, but as her grandfather becomes more forgetful, she finds no way back home from the grocery store and even knows her surroundings. Finally, he cannot take care of himself and do his daily chores. The above-mentioned biography describes a group of brain diseases that we call dementia. These diseases disrupt different parts of the brain and impair one's memory, judgment, reasoning, and planning functions (Weintraub, Wicklund, & Salmon, 2012). Dementia is not a new disease; the earliest writing on this type of disease goes back to the ancient Greek texts. Among the known types of dementia, Alzheimer's disease is more common than others. Alzheimer's usually occurs at an early age. About 10 percent of people over the age of 65 have Alzheimer's. There is also a type of Alzheimer's disease that is less common and occurs at an earlier age. Alzheimer's has a slow and dormant onset. But gradually the person loses the ability to remember recent events. As the disease progresses, the person's disability goes beyond memory and language, orientation, and emotions are also involved. In Alzheimer's disease, the brain's suprabasal area, called the cortex, shrinks, resulting in impaired thinking, planning, and memory functions. This shrinkage is more severe in an area called the hippocampus that is responsible for creating new memories (Summers & Saunders, 2012).

NEUROPSYCHOLOGICAL FUNCTIONING IN SCHIZOPHRENIA

Schizophrenia is one of the most common serious mental disorders and occurs in about 1% of the world population but its underlying nature has not yet been elucidated and is therefore sometimes referred to as a syndrome, i.e., a group of schizophrenia or as in the fifth edition of the Diagnostic Manuscript And the statistic of mental disorders has been described, it's called the schizophrenia spectrum. Although schizophrenia is described as a single disease, it is probably composed of a group of disorders that have heterogeneous etiology and include patients whose clinical manifestations, therapeutic response, and course of the disease are not the same (Kaplan, 2016).

In these patients, there is no unity between thoughts and feelings. Today, psychiatric patients are classified into two distinct morphs, each with different causes. The first form is characterized by an acute onset and with positive symptoms such as hallucinations, delusions, thought disorders (disordered thinking, and irrational thinking), behavioral disorders, and responds well to medication. Conversely, in the latter, the course of the disease is chronic and is accompanied by negative symptoms such as lack of motivation, mental slowness, and avoidance, response to drug therapy in these patients is not appropriate and structural changes in the brain such as ventricular dilatation are seen (Schaefer et al., 2019; Ye, Zhan, Xiao, Sha, & Zhang, 2018).

So far, some researches in the form of books and articles have examined the physiology of neuropsychological function in individuals. For example, according to the neurodevelopmental hypothesis of schizophrenia, etiologic and pathogenic factors begin before the formal onset of the disease and during pregnancy and disrupt normal growth. These subtle early changes in some neurons, glia cells, and circuits may make a person vulnerable to subsequent growth factors and eventually lead to scarring. It is evident that schizophrenia is a multifactorial disorder and both environmental and genetic factors are involved. In clinical trials using risk assessment, some relevant factors have been identified, including birth and prenatal complications (hypoxia, infection, exposure to toxic substances or substances), family history, body deformity, especially structures of neuronal origin and defects. These risk factors may affect current growth processes such as axonal and dendritic experience-dependent production, programmed cell death, myelination, and synaptic pruning.

In imaging and pathological studies, structural abnormalities have been identified at the time of disease manifestation, including small frontal cortex and hippocampus, and abnormal enlargement, indicating abnormal growth. Structural nerve imaging supports the conclusion that the hippocampus in schizophrenia is significantly smaller and maybe up to 5% smaller. In people who are more severely affected, more areas are affected and changes are greater. In some cases, over time, ventricular enlargement and atrophy of the cortical gray matter increase. These ongoing progressive changes should lead us to reconsider the potential role of active demise in schizophrenia, whether due to the disease itself or its consequences, such as stress or drug treatment.

Comparison of the synchrony of twins in one egg and two eggs in terms of schizophrenia confirms the role of both genetic and environmental factors in this disorder. In single-twin eggs, only 40 to 50 percent of all twins are infected, indicating that genetic nature alone does not mean disease and the fetal environment. Neurological, pharmacological, and pathological imaging studies show that some genetic factors are associated with susceptibility to secondary aggression, such as prenatal or viral infection. This model is consistent with findings from imaging studies showing that hippocampal volume decreased in both infected and uninfected egg twins.

The frontal lobe is one of the most important parts of the brain that is involved in neuroscience function. Much research has pointed to the relationship between the frontal lobe and executive functions. The frontal lobe, which accounts for about one-third of the brain's volume, plays an important role in thoughts, emotions, behaviors, reasoning, problem-solving, attentiveness, judgment, creativity, awareness, and impulse control. Other functions of the frontal lobe include simple and complex motor skills and motor inhibition (Schoenberg & Scott, 2011).

The results of studies on twins and offspring suggest that the disorder can be genetically caused. The matching rate of twins in one egg is usually five times that of twins. One of the hereditary traits may be due to a deficiency in the immune system that disrupts the functioning of the brain and consequently damages brain tissue. According to the fitness hypothesis, some people have schizophrenia genes that appear in the right environment. Also, schizophrenia can be caused by non-genetic factors such as fetal and birth injuries (Picchioni et al., 2017; van Haren & Psychiatry, 2017).

One of the important hypotheses about schizophrenia is the dopamine hypothesis, which suggests that schizophrenia is caused by the high activity of lateral and subcortical dopaminergic cells. According to this hypothesis, schizophrenia is caused by over-activity of dopaminergic synapses, and this occurs in two ways: 1- Dopaminergic cells may be activated and release more dopamine than usual and postsynaptic dopamine receptors are more sensitive in the brain of affected individuals;

Another is that cells that stimulate dopaminergic cells become overactive or cells that inhibit them become less active. Although there is no strong evidence to support the hypothesis of dopamine, researchers consider the role of dopamine in the development of this important mental disorder (O. D. Howes & Kapur, 2009; Stahl, 2018).

Most people with schizophrenia show neurological symptoms that indicate brain damage. Symptoms include abnormal facial movements, slow or fast blinking, glare, avoiding eye contact, lack of blinking in response to the gentle forehead, eye deviation, inability to move eyes without head movement, and reactions. These symptoms suggest that schizophrenia may be associated with some kind of brain injury (Fong, Ho, Wan, & Au-Yeung, 2017; López et al., 2016).

The results of computed tomography and magnetic resonance imaging studies of patients with schizophrenia show that the relative size of their lateral ventricles is twice that of normal subjects. Larger ventricles are probably due to a lack of brain tissue. Also, computed tomography of 54 patients showed that parts of their forehead, frontal-temporal, and hypothalamic tissues were missing. Also, the findings of Anderson (1992) showed that the brain of many schizophrenia patients has abnormalities in the corpus callosum and the hippocampus. Suddath concluded that twin magnetic resonance imaging showed that patients with schizophrenia had larger lateral ventricles and third ventricles, and the twin hippocampus was smaller than normal and had gray matter volume. Their left is reduced (Anderson, 1992; Suddath, Christison, Torrey, Casanova, & Weinberger, 1990).

The complexity of schizophrenia disorder has led to various hypotheses. One of the common hypotheses is neuropsychological malfunctions. On the other hand, schizophrenia and other severe mental illnesses are increasingly being considered as neurocognitive disorders, and deficits in the neuropsychological and neurocognitive functions are considered the central characteristic of schizophrenia. People with schizophrenia have also shown abnormalities in various neurological and executive functions in a variety of neurological tests. Studies in memory, response inhibition, and cognitive flexibility, for example, have shown that patients with schizophrenia have impaired memory, response inhibition, and cognitive flexibility.

One explanation for a defect in inhibition is orbitofrontal cortex lesions that impair response inhibition, and neuroimaging studies have shown that activity in the orbitofrontal cortex intensifies in tasks that require behavior suppression. The orbitofrontal cortex acts as one of the important regions of the prefrontal cortex that sends the information needed to inhibit the response to the lower brain areas. Running during assignments requires behavior offsets, the ability to be reversible and to delay momentum. Many studies show that the orbitofrontal cortex is a type of inhibitory signal that provides for the abolition or modulation of behavioral responsiveness when control is required for accurate performance. Imaging studies have shown strong signals generated by the orbitofrontal cortex in experiments in which subjects require response inhibition.

Although neuro-cognitive deficits are not yet recognized as diagnostic criteria for schizophrenia, they are still considered as one of the major features of schizophrenia. One of the key abilities in executive-cognitive functions is cognitive flexibility. Cognitive flexibility is the ability to adapt quickly to changing environmental demands, prioritize according to the needs of the environment, and adapt to changes with new and different perspectives. Cognitive flexibility is crucial for creativity, learning, and directing attention and is closely linked to social cognition and interpersonal relationships (Bolea, 2010). There is also a defect in cognitive flexibility during the first course of schizophrenia and maybe one of the inherent features of schizophrenia. This finding supports the neurodevelopmental origin of schizophrenia. The underlying mechanisms of cognitive flexibility have been explored and identified using various methods. The study, using functional magnetic resonance imaging (fMRI), has shown areas of the brain involved in cognitive flexibility that include the prefrontal cortex, basal ganglia, anterior cingulate cortex, and posterior parietal cortex (Caletti et al., 2013).

Neurological-cognitive deficits indicate that there is a disorder in the prefrontal cortex in schizophrenia; these include difficulty in initiating a voluntary response, inability to shift and shift attention and cognitive parameters, inhibition of tissue response inappropriate, and retention of working memory information. There are also qualitative similarities in the neuropsychological deficits of schizophrenic and depressed patients, which have been proven through deficits in neurological and executive functions across these disorders (Orellana & Slachevsky, 2013). However, the severity of neurological and neurological deficits in these disorders varies, with the most common in schizophrenic patients and fewer reported in patients with major depressive disorder. Regarding the neurophysiological abnormalities of most schizophrenic patients than depressed patients due to the neurodevelopmental hypothesis of schizophrenia, it can be said that schizophrenia is perceived as an organic disease during the developmental process and its symptoms are mainly cognitive and cognitive. It is damaged, it gradually appears, so as one's cognitive function develops, it gradually declines. Another hypothesis in the explanation of lower neuropsychological function in schizophrenic patients is that the nature of schizophrenia disorder leads to impaired neuropsychological ability and function in schizophrenic patients (Frith, 2014).

IMPROVING NEUROPSYCHOLOGICAL FUNCTIONING IN SCHIZOPHRENIA

After reviewing the neuropsychology of schizophrenia disorder and its evaluation methods, it is best to discuss ways to improve the neurological function of these patients. So far, neuroscientists have been assessing the neurodevelopmental function of individuals and there has been little effort to improve and improve these functions, but the role of neurodevelopmental improvement in individuals with schizophrenia should be highlighted in the future. One effective way is for neuroscientists to refer to psychiatrists, counselors, and caregivers after evaluating schizophrenia patients for rehabilitation.

Case studies of case studies and group therapy have shown that short-term interventions can improve cognitive and executive functioning of individuals. These short-term interventions should be put together and form a robust treatment protocol to provide more effective and effective assistance to people with neurodevelopmental disorders. Some researchers have shown that cognitive-behavioral therapy can improve attention and executive ability in ADHD adults (Rapport, Orban, Kofler, & Friedman, 2013). The researchers have suggested that this treatment may also be applied to other patients who have problems with neuropsychological functions. Cognitive-behavioral therapy focuses on enhancing a variety of executive functions, such as problem-planning and problem solving, and thus can improve patients' executive functions. Exercise can also improve the cognitive and executive function of patients. In a meta-analysis study, Kolkomb and Kramer showed that exercise had a significant effect on executive performance. Specific recommendations for enhancing executive functioning are based on a variety of factors such as neurological conditions, co-morbidities, and severity of cognitive impairment, impaired awareness, age, and social support (Randolph, 2018).

We can divide compensation strategies to improve executive performance into two categories: external or environmental strategies and internal strategies. Salberg and Meter (2001) used external and internal strategies to enhance executive functions, to create a bridge between theory and practice. They first pointed to the importance of the physical and psychological environment of individuals. Being neat and tidy as well as keeping things neat and tidy are examples of the physical environment. Healthy eating, regular sleep schedule, and adherence to drug therapy are examples of the psychological environment (Randolph, 2018).

Rehabilitation

Rehabilitation is one of the most important treatments for brain damage. The goal of rehabilitation is to return the patient to a normal level of activity so that the patient can make the most of their remaining abilities through planned activities (Bellack, Gold, & Buchanan, 1999).

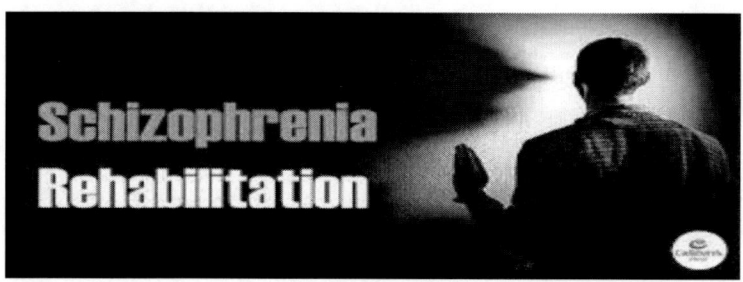

The majority of psychiatric patients who require long-term hospitalization and rehabilitation are those with schizophrenia. Many of these patients have reached the age of onset with their illness, and in addition to the complications of schizophrenia, they also have deficiencies and diseases caused by aging. Unlike previous decades, when there was no effective treatment for schizophrenia, immediate diagnosis and timely treatment with effective drugs can prevent prevention and treatment, and dramatically improve the quality of life for patients and their caregivers. Currently, the artificial classification of schizophrenic patients is not valid for acute and chronic types, and it is recommended, instead of setting up special hospitals for psychiatric patients to exclude patients from the community. Better access to health care and rehabilitation than the psychological and social consequences of staying in private psychiatric hospitals (Liberman, 1986).

Daycare clients include those who have been suffering from neuroscience such as schizophrenia for years, whose mental capacity includes cognitive abilities (memory, the concentration of thought, ability to plan and make decisions, etc.) and skills. Social problems (such as connecting with others, solving current issues in the community, using urban services, commuting in the city, etc.) have been impaired. These disabilities lead to further isolation and isolation of the patient from society. Increasing isolation results in a further decline in patients' mental capacity. This vicious circle will not allow the patient to gradually acquire the necessary abilities or lose them if they are acquired in previous years. The latter is more likely to be the case if the disease starts at an older age, for example, at age 6.

For the treatment of the patient, first of all, it is necessary to take treatment such as hospitalization (in case of the acute phase of illness), medication, or outpatient treatment. This treatment can control and eliminate the acute symptoms of the disease. After the acute phase of the illness, which takes one to three months, the treatment enters a new phase, called rehabilitation. The same procedure briefly described in the first paragraph.

Cognitive, behavioral, and social skills are not something that can be improved or improved by medicine. These require services that are known as rehabilitation or mental rehabilitation. This is a long and time-consuming phase and may sometimes last until the end of life.

In most mental health centers for schizophrenia patients do the following:

- Acquire social skills. It is clear that this skill will be the basis of working in society and among the people after acquiring the necessary knowledge. The use of the subway, public and recreational areas such as the cinema, the park, and the restaurant are among the few activities that can be adjusted and implemented in terms of center capacity and patients per month (Lysaker, Bell, Zito, Bioty, & Disease, 1995).
- Cognitive skills. Practicing and Mobilizing Different Parts of the Brain With paper and computer exercises, one of the measures that are offered to each patient is to stimulate different parts of the brain, especially the frontal part (Krabbendam & Aleman, 2003).
- Exercise and stretching exercises and fine-grained exercises to correct muscular dysfunction and correct organ dysfunctions (Vancampfort et al., 2012).
- Teaching the patient, the causes and symptoms, and methods of preventing the patient from recurring to the patient and his or her family, with the aim of facilitating acceptance of the disease and removing the negative view of the patient and the illness (Chan, Lee, & Chan, 2007).

- Personal health education, which is one of the hallmarks of this category of diseases (Pekkala & Merinder, 2002).
- Monitoring the patient's mental health status and family coordination and referral to a specialist if needed (Wing, Moss, Rabin, & George, 2012).
- Acquiring communication skills and socializing. Regular sessions are held each week to practice social skills, personal communication, family practice, and the like, according to the available scientific resources each week. Attempts are made to provide training videos to the participants in the sessions to expedite the modification of behaviors and to use role-playing techniques by center experts (Dickinson, Bellack, & Gold, 2006).
- Acquire professional skills. Depending on their talents, they are assigned to work, carpet weaving and painting, and, after undergoing the introductory steps, are introduced to a professional technical organization to pursue a vocational training phase in order to gain the necessary skills there (Heinssen, Liberman, & Kopelowicz, 2000).
- Holding educational meetings with families. In order to continue these activities at home, the family must also be familiar with the activities at the center for patients and at home. Also, get the necessary education about the illness and meet with each other and share experiences with other families (Dixon, Adams, & Lucksted, 2000; W. R. McFarlane, Dixon, Lukens, Lucksted, & therapy, 2003).

In this section, we have tried to summarize some of the most important psychological measures for schizophrenia patients. These include drug therapy, occupational therapy, group therapy, family therapy, group therapy and cognitive behavioral therapy, electric shock treatment, hospitalization, occupational rehabilitation, cognitive rehabilitation, follow-up social therapy, acceptance therapy, and commitment.

1. Medication

Schizophrenia requires lifelong treatment, even when symptoms have resolved. Medication and psychotherapy can help control the disease. In some cases, hospitalization may be required. An experienced psychiatrist in the treatment of schizophrenia usually guides the treatment process. The psychiatrist also works with a medical team, which may include a psychologist, social worker, psychiatric nurse, and possibly a manager to coordinate care activities (Lacro, Dunn, Dolder, Leckband, & Jeste, 2002).

With such support, determination, and awareness, a person with schizophrenia can learn how to cope and live with their condition. But the stability associated with this disorder means adherence to a regulated treatment plan between the individual and the physician and maintaining the balance provided by the medication and treatment. Sudden cessation of treatment often results in the return of symptoms and then gradual improvement will continue as treatment continues (Higashi et al., 2013).

Medications are the cornerstone of schizophrenia treatment, and antipsychotics are the most common prescription drugs. These drugs control symptoms by affecting the neurotransmitter dopamine (Thieda, Beard, Richter, & Kane, 2003).

The purpose of treatment with antipsychotics is to effectively control the signs and symptoms with the lowest possible dose. The psychiatrist may use different medications and doses or a combination of medications over time to achieve the desired results. Other drugs, such as antidepressants or anxiolytics, may also be effective. Symptom recovery can take several weeks (Lieberman et al., 2005).

Because the drugs used for schizophrenia can cause serious side effects, people with schizophrenia may not be willing to take them. The willingness and willingness to cooperate for treatment can influence the choice of medication. For example, a person who is constantly resisting medication may need to be given injection instead of a pill. Talk to your doctor about the benefits and side effects of any prescription drug.

The following are common prescription drugs:

1. First Generation Anti-Psychotic Drugs (Leucht et al., 2009):
   First-generation antipsychotics have frequent and potentially significant side effects, including the likelihood of a motor disorder (late-onset motility) that may not be reversible. These include:

   - Chloroformazine
   - Fluphenazine
   - Haloperidol
   - Perphenazine

   These antipsychotics are often cheaper than the second generation, especially the generic one, which can be an important factor if long-term treatment is needed.

2. Second Generation Antipsychotic Drugs (Rummel-Kluge et al., 2010):

   These newer second-generation drugs are generally preferred because they are less susceptible to side effects than the first generation. These include:

   - Aripiprazine
   - Asenapine
   - Piperazole
   - Cariprazine
   - Clozapine
   - Iloperidone
   - Lorazidone
   - Olanzapine
   - Quetiapine
   - Polypyridone
   - Risperidone

- Ziprasidone

2. Therapeutic Work

Studies have shown that occupational therapy is one of the important elements in the successful treatment of schizophrenia and other severe cognitive disorders. In addition to psychiatrists, psychologists, and social workers, occupational therapy also helps mentally ill people in work and social settings and enhances their confidence and independence. Occupational therapy with medication, skills training, and other services helps patients to return to the community (Hewitt & Coffey, 2005).

The work of therapists working with schizophrenic patients improves their self-esteem, social relationships, and leisure activities. Specialists in neurosurgical rehabilitation centers reduce the symptoms of schizophrenia and help improve their treatment.

Throughout life, therapeutic work helps patients to achieve the things they want and need through daily activities as therapeutic activities. Occupational therapists help people of all ages improve their health and lead a good life, and avoid injury, illness, and problems.

Common practices in occupational therapy (Stapleton & McBrearty, 2009) include:

- Helping patients attend social situations
- Helping affected people to improve and regain skills
- Support for adults with physical and cognitive changes.

Occupational Therapy Services (Case-Smith, 2003) include:

- Comprehensive assessment of patients' living and other living environments (such as workplaces)
- An individual assessment, during which the patient, the patient's family, and the occupational therapist determine the individual's therapeutic goals.
- Advice on using the equipment and learning how to use it
- Guidance and training for family members and therapists

- Partnerships to enhance the patient's ability to perform daily activities and achieve goals
- Evaluate results to ensure goals are achieved or changed in the partnership program

Characteristics of occupational therapy behaviors (Mills & Millsteed, 2002) are:

- Dysfunction: False judgment, lack of organization
- Hostility: Negative attitude, aggression
- Child behavior: Lack of independence, asking for help
- Socialism: Waiting for rejection, withdrawal
- Pathological Emotional Response: Inattention, Exaggerated and Inappropriate Responses

Specific occupational therapy applications (Kuhaneck & Watling, 2015) include:

- Development and development of interpersonal relationships
- Supporting the patient to recognize themselves as a person with rights, needs, personal identity and values
- The patient must feel accepted by others; the environment must accept him and accept him as he is.
- Coordination with the patient: Talk to the patient as slowly as you need to and move with him or her, do not disturb the patient by sudden movement or speech.
- Give the patient enough time to get things done and help them get ready.
- Make it easy for the patient to communicate: Use non-verbal ways to communicate, try to talk to the patient at the same level, and use the words he or she uses.
- Avoid excessive, overbearing, and overbearing behavior.

- The patient should be supported and encouraged when trying to gain independence.

Occupational Therapists

Occupational therapists have a general view. One of the features of their perspective is the focus on adapting to the environment, and the patient is an integral part of the treatment group. An occupational therapist can identify the strengths and problems of a patient's life, such as dressing or shopping, and helping the patient find workable solutions to get things done. Specialists work with the patient to identify goals that help the patient gain and increase their independence by using different methods, changing the environment, and using new equipment (Curtin & Fossey, 2007).

Occupational Therapy in Schizophrenia

People with schizophrenia have problems with social and cognitive functioning, self-care, residual negative symptoms, high rates of unemployment, and social deprivation. The goal is to treat, treat, and rehabilitate people with severe mental disorders (Morris, Reid, & Spencer, 2018).

The goals of occupational therapy for schizophrenic patients include:

- Improved communication with the real world
- Strengthen your individual self
- Provide a way out for hostility
- Reduce dependency
- Raising patient standards and values
- Improvement of motor and cognitive abilities
- Improve your self-care

Proper Activities

Appropriate activities are activities that provide the opportunity for the patient to create real or artificial satisfaction and to meet the needs of the patient, depending on the extent of improvement.

Satisfactory oral activities such as eating, biting, chewing, dying, etc.

- Prepare and eat food
- Watch and collect food images
- Soap bubbles die, chew gum or die on musical instruments

Pleasant works activities such as disposal management, maintenance activities, etc.

- gardening, soil preparation, and flowering
- Wash and clean clothes, aisles, dishes, and utensils
- Garbage collection, rubbish and foot cleaning

Activities that enhance sensory, perceptual, and motor coordination include:

- Integrated muscle activity
- Balanced handling and walking

Activities that make the patient autonomous and stop improving as the patient improves include:

- Help and help the patient
- Not expecting the patient to plan and start work, avoiding decisions beyond the patient's ability

Activities that enhance one's self-esteem, self-esteem, sense of self-worth, and standards of value include:

- Creating a sense of individual identity: Designing individual projects for the patient's personal use
- Increasing one's self-development: taking care of one's self, creating one's own beauty, ensuring one's successful endeavor based on one's abilities
- Encourage and respect one's feelings and views about activities

Activities that help release hostility are:

- Using non-aggressive activities: By increasing patient tolerance, performing aggressive activities such as hammering, woodworking.

Activities that provide opportunities to test and experience reality such as:

- Perform activities that increase contact with reality.
- Activities that provide the opportunity to adjust to reality.

Activities that allow the patient to experience a sense of belonging, such as:

- Sharing emotions and shared experiences
- Participate in user group activities

Activities that provide opportunities for social interaction for the patient, such as:

- The symbolic expression of emotion
- Successes that give rise to desirable criticism.

Increase trading like:

- Shared use of equipment
- Do things in turn
- Helping others
- Performing group projects

3. Family Therapy

Family therapy, sometimes called family-centered therapy or family system therapy, is a psychological therapy that works to change relationships within families in order to help them cope with a range of problems. Family therapy is a form of counseling that helps you and your family resolve your problems when they occur. This treatment usually includes education about and treatment for schizophrenia. Family therapy is important because your family can play a key role in supporting you if you have schizophrenia (Smerud & Rosenfarb, 2011).

Family therapy can significantly reduce the rate of return for a person with schizophrenia. In stressful families, patients with schizophrenia have a 1–5% return rate in the first year after hospital discharge under standard care. Supportive family therapy can reduce this rate of return to less than 1%. This treatment encourages the family to hold a family meeting whenever there is a problem to determine the main nature of the problem after the discussion, consider alternative solutions, and select and implement the best solution agreed.

Family therapy or family counseling is done to address specific problems that affect the family's mental health, such as major life changes or other mental illnesses. Family interventions have been shown to reduce the rate of relapse and the need for hospitalization in patients with schizophrenia. Our specialists at the Neurological Rehabilitation Center provide family services to reduce the symptoms of schizophrenia (W. R. J. F. P. McFarlane, 2016).

Family Therapy helps families find productive ways to help each other. Due to its flexibility, this type of treatment is useful in a wide range of different diseases. This treatment can be helpful in resolving childhood and adolescence problems, including behavioral and mood disorders, eating disorders, substance abuse, and mental conditions, as well as couples who have problems. Family therapy is a possible treatment for several diseases, including serious mental illnesses such as depression and schizophrenia, and is usually administered in family groups, but will sometimes include working with individuals individually or, if necessary, having individual meetings together with a set of family referrals. Family therapy may also include social networks around families (Friedlander, Escudero, Heatherington, & Diamond, 2011).

Family therapy is based on two principles:

- Many diseases worsen if the family functions improperly.
- Close family relationships are often the most important support a person has and are therefore very important in any long-term treatment.

Family therapy can be defined as a psychological treatment that focuses on:

- Changing the way family members interact
- Improving family functioning as a unit
- Improving the performance of individuals in the family

The effect of Family Therapy

Family therapy seems to be used to improve various conditions. There is good evidence that family therapy is very useful in the following childhood and adolescent diseases:

- Behavioral disorders
- Substance abuse
- Eating Disorders (Like Anorexia)

- Behavioral disorders (including inattention and hyperactivity)

In adults, family therapy has been helpful in:

- Mental disorders (including schizophrenia) (W. R. McFarlane et al., 2003)
- mood disorders (including depression and bipolar disorder (Diamond et al., 2010; Lauder, Berk, Castle, Dodd, & Berk, 2010)
- Drug use (Rowe & therapy, 2012)
- Eating disorders (Couturier, Kimber, & Szatmari, 2013)
- Anxiety Disorders (S. Schneider et al., 2013)
- Obsessive-Compulsive Disorders (Lebowitz, Panza, Su, & Bloch, 2012)

There are various types of family therapy that can often be used together. These include:

- *Mental education*: This treatment focuses on educating the family about the disease to change any negative (and possibly wrong) perceptions that family members may have about the disease.
- *Training in coping skills*
- *Behavioral models*: These models focus on teaching parents about positive and negative reinforcement to help them deal with child behavior problems.
- *Systemic Models*: Such models believe that adverse family relationships often worsen the disease and thus improve family relationships and improve symptoms.
- *Structural Family Therapy*: This type of treatment focuses on restoring proper family structure and organization.
- *Post-Milan Family Therapy*: This treatment is based on communication between family members.

- *Solution-Focused Therapy*: This method emphasizes identifying each family member's strengths and then using these strengths to help solve problems.

These are just some of the different ways that family therapy can be used to overcome any family or individual problems that family members experience.

The Benefits of Family Therapy for Schizophrenia

Patients with schizophrenia often come from family groups with a high level of hostility or disapproval. For this reason, family therapy has long been suggested as a possible treatment for schizophrenia.

There is currently extensive evidence for the use of family therapy to improve schizophrenia. The different types of family therapy that are used include more traditional psychological education and communication improvement as well as newer approaches including motivational interviewing, crisis management treatment, and even relaxation therapy. The number and type of family therapy sessions required will vary depending on the individual and family.

Family therapy has been shown to reduce symptoms and can also reduce the number of times the patient should be hospitalized. Family therapy can also be helpful in reducing the isolation and social isolation that many people with schizophrenia suffer from. Another benefit of family therapy is that most people who receive this treatment use their medication more regularly, resulting in fewer symptoms and a better quality of life.

Family therapy is not a quick and easy solution and it takes time and effort for the desired outcome. Families undergoing family therapy should be aware that family therapy involves formal meetings and work at home, where new learned skills and techniques must be practiced daily, on a daily basis. The number of formal meetings depends largely on illness and family activity.

Usually, between 1 and 2 sessions are required. Meetings usually take between 1 minute and 1 hour. Treatment sessions often include a family specialist who meets with several family members at the same time (this will directly resolve any problems between family members and allow the therapist to assess the family carefully). There are also individual meetings and possibly meetings with more family members or other important friends.

Although there is good evidence that family therapy is a very useful tool, many people are concerned about the high costs of family therapy. However, recent analyzes show that family therapy can significantly reduce the cost of medical care. This is because if family therapy works, the individual (and his or her family) will use less medical care services (including referrals, medications, etc.) and overall savings will be sought for both the family and the wider community.

Family therapy does not automatically solve the family's internal problems or resolve an unpleasant situation. But it can help you and your family members understand each other better and provide you with the skills to deal with challenging situations more effectively. It can also help the family develop a sense of solidarity.

If family therapy is not managed properly by a well-trained counselor, it can worsen some of the problems. If this treatment is stopped too early, it may not solve the problems well enough. If a family member refuses to participate, it may lose its effect.

4. Group Therapy

Group therapy and drug therapy together, especially in patients with schizophrenia, will have relatively better outcomes than mere drug therapy. When group therapy focuses on real-life plans, problems, and relationships, as well as occupational and social laws and relationships, and combines drug therapy and side effects or some practical hobbies or work activities; and the positive increases. This type of supportive group therapy can be especially beneficial in reducing social isolation and increasing reality testing.

If you are thinking about psychotherapy, there are several options available to you, one of which is group therapy. Depending on the nature of your problem, group therapy can be a good choice to address your problem and make a positive difference in your life. Group therapy can be very effective in treating schizophrenia. Our specialists at the Neurophysiological Rehabilitation Center can give you more information about the treatment group and how it can affect your mental illness.

The goals of group therapy are:

- Helping patients to identify abnormal behaviors
- Solve emotional problems through feedback and then improve people's ability to overcome difficult problems
- Providing a supportive environment for participants

Joining a group of strangers and strangers may seem scary at first, but group therapy has benefits that individual treatment lacks. In fact, psychologists say group members are almost always amazed at how great the group experience can be.

Groups can be seen as a supportive and local network of ideas. Other members of the group often help you express ideas to improve a difficult situation or life's challenges and hold you accountable along the way.

In most cases, talking and listening to others can help you judge your problems better and more correctly. Many people experience mental health problems, but few can easily talk about their problems to others who are not well aware of it. Often times you may feel that you are the only one to deal with these problems, but it is not. Listening to others talk about what you have been through and what they have experienced can relieve you and show you that you are not alone.

Another important advantage of group therapy is its diversity. People have different personalities and backgrounds and look at the situation from different angles. By seeing how other people eliminate problems and make positive changes, you can discover a range of strategies to deal with your problems (Orfanos, Banks, Priebe, & Psychosomatics, 2015).

Who Needs Group Therapy?

- Communication problems
- Some personality disorders
- Schizophrenia
- Depression
- Anxiety and Agoraphobia and Obsessive-Compulsive Disorder (OCD)
- More specific groups, such as bullying, women who have been sexually abused.

Principles and Principles of Treatment

Key therapeutic principles (Orfanos et al., 2015) derived from the self-assessments of individuals attending group therapy courses are:

- *Induce Hope*: Members of a group are at different stages of the treatment process. Seeing those who are struggling or recovering gives hope to those at the beginning of the treatment process.
- *Generality*: Being a member of a group of people who have all gone through the same experience helps them to know that what they have experienced in public and that they are not alone.
- *Exchange of information*: Group members can help each other by sharing their information.
- *Friendship*: Group members can share their strengths with each other and help other members of the group to enhance their self-esteem and confidence.
- *Repeating the initial family group as a modifier*: The treatment group is in some ways very similar to a family. In one group, each member can explore childhood experiences that have contributed to his or her personality and behavior. They can also learn to avoid behaviors that are real, destructive, and ineffective in real life.
- *Expanding Socialization Techniques*: The group environment is a great place to practice new behaviors. It's a safe and supportive

environment, allowing team members to test and error without fear of failure.
- *Imitation Behavior*: Individuals can pattern other behaviors in their group or observe and imitate therapist behavior.
- *Interpersonal learning*: Group members can gain a better understanding of themselves by interacting with others and receiving feedback from the therapist and therapist.
- *Group cohesion*: Because members of a group are united in one goal, members of the group will have a sense of belonging and acceptance.
- *Emotional evacuation*: Sharing experiences and emotions with a group of people can help relieve pain, guilt, or stress.
- *Existential Factors*: When you work in a group, the group supports and guides you, the group therapist helps group members find out that they are responsible for their lives, actions, and choices.

How Does Group Therapy Work?

Groups can be as small as three or four people, but group therapy sessions are often about 1 to 4 people (although there may be more participants). Group members usually meet once or twice a week for one or two hours.

The minimum number of group sessions is usually 3 times, but one-year sessions are more common. These sessions can also be open or closed. In open sessions, new participants can be accepted into the group at any time. In a closed group, only a core group of members is invited to attend.

In many cases, the group comes together in a room where the chairs are arranged in a large circle and each member can see the other members of the group. The meeting may begin by introducing the group members themselves and explaining why they are in the treatment group. Members may describe their experiences and developments from the previous meeting to date.

The exact way in which the meetings are run depends largely on the goals of the group and the therapist's approach. Some therapists may pursue a more open conversation style, with each member attending the meeting in a way that suits them best.

This is a very controversial issue. Further studies should be conducted to compare group therapy with other treatments. Group therapy, while helping some people, can have negative effects on others. For example, the severity of existing symptoms or the appearance of new symptoms. The causes of treatment failure can be influenced by several factors, such as the difficult and inappropriate relationship between the patient and the therapist.

5. Cognitive Behavioral Therapy

Cognitive-behavioral therapy in patients with schizophrenia was initially developed to provide additional treatments for residual symptoms based on the principles and strategies of intervention previously developed for anxiety and depression. About 1% of psychiatric patients with persistent positive and negative symptoms do not need medication treatment, even if they are compatible with prescription medications. However, despite the introduction of unusual antipsychotics, patient compliance with the drug is still a major problem. Studies have shown that 4% of outpatient and inpatient patients have stopped their treatment.

Cognitive-behavioral therapy in schizophrenia patients is currently recognized as an effective intervention for schizophrenia in clinical guidelines. Despite available evidence that side effects are absent, public access to this treatment in the community remains limited and low (Sarin, Wallin, & Widerlöv, 2011).

Cognitive-Behavioral Therapy is a goal-based approach to solving the problem of mental illness, especially in schizophrenia patients, with the goal of changing the patterns of thinking or behavior that are behind people's problems and changing their feelings.

Cognitive-behavioral therapy in schizophrenia patients is a common type of speech therapy (psychotherapy). You talk to a psychologist or psychotherapist in a structured way and with a specific number of sessions.

This will help you identify the wrong or negative thinking so you can see the challenging situations more clearly and respond in a more effective way. Cognitive-behavioral therapy can be a very useful tool in the treatment of mental disorders such as schizophrenia, depression, post-traumatic stress disorder, or an eating disorder, but not everyone who benefits from cognitive behavioral therapy in schizophrenic patients may necessarily have complete mental health. This therapy can be an effective tool to help anyone learn how to manage stressful life situations (Burns, Erickson, & Brenner, 2014).

The Benefits of Cognitive Behavioral Therapy in Schizophrenia Patients (Burns et al., 2014)

Cognitive-behavioral therapy in schizophrenia patients can also be effective in treating some mental health problems, but may not be effective for everyone. Some of the benefits of cognitive-behavioral therapy in schizophrenia include:

- It may be helpful in cases where the drug alone does not work.
- Completes in a relatively shorter period than other speech therapies.
- The highly organized nature of cognitive-behavioral therapy in schizophrenia patients means it can be presented in a variety of formats, including in groups, tutorials, and computer programs.
- It teaches you useful and practical strategies that can be used in everyday life, even after treatment is completed.

Work Process (Burns et al., 2014)

The treatment techniques used for patients with schizophrenia are based on the general principles of cognitive-behavioral therapy. Links between thoughts, feelings, and actions are created in a friendly and receptive environment. Programs are prescribed and used but are generally more flexible than traditional cognitive behavioral therapy. Psychotherapy usually proceeds as follows.

Assessment

The psychologist allows the patient to express his thoughts about his experiences while the therapist listens fully to the patient and evaluates him. Specific and general scales are used to monitor patient progress and the results are shared with the patient. Diagrams and cases can be useful, especially for patients with a chaotic lifestyle. Causes of current symptoms and findings are also discussed with the patient, and during treatment with new information, the patient's records and information will be more complete (Burns et al., 2014).

Interaction Stage

Initially, the therapist clearly states the method and purpose of treatment, including a safe and general method for examining the causes of anxiety. The use of Socratic questionnaires has been emphasized during treatment. These questions are guided by the discovery process in order to discover one understands of one's own situation and the appropriate ways to respond to it. The psychologist strives to understand and empathize with the patient's unique vision and feelings and is always flexible in dealing with the patient. A stress vulnerability model is used so that the patient can understand that vulnerability is a dynamic concept that can be influenced by many factors such as life events, coping mechanisms, or physical illnesses. The therapist emphasizes that she does not have all the answers for the patient, but can help her more if they interact and work together. General factors of treatment, such as generating intimacy, sincerity, humor, and empathy, are as valuable as other therapies.

The stages of cognitive-behavioral therapy in schizophrenia patients (Hofmann et al., 2012) usually include the following:

- Identify difficult and difficult situations and situations in your life. These conditions may include medical conditions, divorce, sadness, anger, or symptoms of mental illness. You and your therapist may take some time to decide what goals you want to focus on.

- Know your thoughts, feelings, and beliefs about these problems. Once you've identified the problems you want to work on, your doctor will encourage you to share your thoughts about them. This sharing of thoughts may include talking to yourself about an experience, your interpretation of a situation, and your beliefs about yourself, your surroundings, and events. Your therapist may suggest that you record your thoughts.
- Identify negative or false thoughts. To help identify patterns of thinking and behavior that may help solve the problem, your doctor may ask you to consider your physical, emotional, and behavioral responses in different situations.
- Change negative or negative thoughts. The therapist encourages you to ask yourself whether your view of a situation is based on reality or a misunderstanding of what is happening! This step may be difficult for you because you probably need to spend a lot of time thinking about your life and yourself. Useful patterns of thought and behavior can become a habit with a practice that does not require much effort to use.

Treatment Duration

Cognitive-behavioral therapy in schizophrenia patients is generally a short-term therapy requiring approximately two to four sessions. You and your therapist can talk to you about the number of sessions that are right for you. Factors affecting the number of treatment sessions are:

- Type of disorder or condition
- Severity of symptoms
- The length of time a person has had symptoms and spent with this condition.
- Speed up one's progress
- The amount of stress the patient has
- How much support do you get from family members and other people?

In general, cognitive-behavioral therapy in schizophrenia patients is of low risk. As this treatment usually relieves the patient's painful feelings and experiences, in some cases the person may feel unwell. You may be upset, crying, angry, or maybe physically weak during a challenging meeting. Some types of cognitive-behavioral therapy in schizophrenia patients, such as the exposure phase, may put you in a situation where you have always wanted to escape. For example, if you are afraid of flying, you may be asked to board a plane. This situation can lead to temporary stress or anxiety. However, working with a skilled expert minimizes any risks. The coping skills you learn can help you manage and overcome negative emotions and fears (Hofmann et al., 2012).

6. Acceptance and Commitment Therapy

Awareness-based acceptance and commitment are used for some conditions, including psychosis. The main purpose of this treatment is not to directly reduce the symptoms of psychosis, but to reduce the suffering of the patient by increasing the tolerability of psychosis symptoms (for example, by increasing self-awareness and acceptance; reducing focus and thereby influencing symptoms and guiding patient focus on core values) (Bach, Hayes, & Gallop, 2012).

7. Follow-Up Social Therapy

Another type of evidence-based treatment for schizophrenia is follow-up social therapy. This treatment is a multidisciplinary team approach that typically includes managers, psychiatrists, social workers, and other mental health practitioners. This approach is an incremental approach to case management where team members work on a case, have frequent contact with the patient (at least once a week), and allow patient access to the community. The goal is to reduce hospital stays and help the patient adapt to life in the community (Lambert et al., 2010).

8. Cognitive Rehabilitation

The goal of short-term cognitive rehabilitation is to improve the cognitive skills required for social and professional functioning in people with schizophrenia, such as using computers and working with paper and pencil. Most of these interventions address the motivational and emotional deficits that are most common in schizophrenia (Hurford, Kalkstein, & Hurford, 2011).

9. Professional Rehabilitation

It focuses on helping people with schizophrenia prepare, find, and maintain jobs. Most people with schizophrenia need some daily support. Many foundations have programs to help people with schizophrenia find work, housing, self-help groups, and critical situations. A manager or person on the treatment team can help find resources. With proper treatment, most people with schizophrenia can control their disease (Bio & Gattaz, 2011; Kluwe-Schiavon, Sanvicente-Vieira, Kristensen, & Grassi-Oliveira, 2013).

10. Hospitalization

During critical periods or during severe symptoms, hospitalization may be required to ensure good health, adequate nutrition, adequate sleep, and basic health (Goldberg et al., 2011).

11. Treatment with Electric Shock

For adults with schizophrenia who do not respond to drug therapy, electric shock therapy may be considered. This treatment can be effective for a person with depression.

People who do not have any mental disorders will continue to learn new social skills for the rest of their lives. It is therefore not a strange thing to expect that people with such diseases will need to receive this type of service long. But the difference is that patients need at least social and cognitive skills to achieve relatively independent living in the community, and the rest will learn the skills they need to live in the community or will sometimes need these services. Thus, we need at least one to two years to acquire these capabilities. It should also be borne in mind that not all patients need the same measure depending on the age of onset of illness, level of education, intelligence, and mental abilities (Zervas, Theleritis, & Soldatos, 2012).

REFERENCES

Afshari, B., Khezrian, K. & Faghihi, A. (2019). Examination and Comparison of Cognitive and Executive Functions in Patients with Schizophrenia and Bipolar Disorders. *J Journal of Isfahan Medical School*. 8. doi:10.22122/jims.v37i320.11149.

Afshari, B., Omidi, A., & Ahmadvand, A. (2019). Effects of Dialectical Behavior Therapy on Executive Functions, Emotion Regulation, and Mindfulness in Bipolar Disorder. 1-9.

Afshari, B., Rasouli-Azad, M., & Ghoreishi, F. (2019). Comparison of original and revised reinforcement sensitivity theory in clinically-stable schizophrenia and bipolar disorder patients. *138*, 321-327.

Anderson, J. R. J. A. j. o. P. (1992). *Automaticity and the ACT* theory.*, *105*(2), 165-180.

Association, A. P. (2013). Diagnostic and statistical manual of mental disorders, (DSM-5®): American Psychiatric Pub. *View Article Google Scholar*.

Bach, P., Hayes, S. C. & Gallop, R. J. B. M. (2012). *Long-term effects of brief acceptance and commitment therapy for psychosis.*, *36*(2), 165-181.

Bain, S. K. & Allin, J. D. J. J. o. P. A. (2005). *Book review: Stanford-binet intelligence scales.*, *23*(1), 87-95.

Bellack, A. S., Gold, J. M. & Buchanan, R. W. J. S. B. (1999). *Cognitive rehabilitation for schizophrenia: problems, prospects, and strategies.*, *25*(2), 257-274.

Bio, D. S. & Gattaz, W. F. J. S. r. (2011). *Vocational rehabilitation improves cognition and negative symptoms in schizophrenia.*, *126*(1-3), 265-269.

Boghi, A., Rasetti, R., Avidano, F., Manzone, C., Orsi, L., D'Agata, F. & Pulvirenti, L. J. N. (2006). *The effect of gender on planning: An fMRI study using the Tower of London task.*, *33*(3), 999-1010.

Bolea, A. S. J. J. o. N. (2010). *Neurofeedback treatment of chronic inpatient schizophrenia.*, *14*(1), 47-54.

Burns, A. M., Erickson, D. H. & Brenner, C. A. J. P. S. (2014). *Cognitive-behavioral therapy for medication-resistant psychosis: a meta-analytic review.*, *65*(7), 874-880.

Caletti, E., Paoli, R. A., Fiorentini, A., Cigliobianco, M., Zugno, E., Serati, M. & Zago, S. J. F. i. h. n. (2013). *Neuropsychology, social cognition and global functioning among bipolar, schizophrenic patients and healthy controls: preliminary data.*, *7*, 661.

Calhoun, V. D., Maciejewski, P. K., Pearlson, G. D. & Kiehl, K. A. J. H. b. m. (2008). *Temporal lobe and "default" hemodynamic brain modes discriminate between schizophrenia and bipolar disorder*, *29*(11), 1265-1275.

Caramazza, A. & Coltheart, M. J. C. N. (2006). *Cognitive neuropsychology twenty years on*, *23*(1), 3-12.

Case-Smith, J. J. A. J. o. O. T. (2003). *Outcomes in hand rehabilitation using occupational therapy services.*, *57*(5), 499-506.

Chan, S. H. W., Lee, S. W. K. & Chan, I. W. M. J. O. t. i. (2007). *TRIP: a psycho-educational programme in Hong Kong for people with schizophrenia.*, *14*(2), 86-98.

Chang, Y. K., Tsai, C. L., Hung, T. M., So, E. C., Chen, F. T., Etnier, J. L. J. J. o. S. & Psychology, E. (2011). *Effects of acute exercise on executive function: a study with a Tower of London Task.*, *33*(6), 847-865.

Chou, P. H., Tang, K. T., Chen, Y. H., Sun, C. W., Huang, C. M. & Chen, D. Y. J. J. o. C. N. (2018). *Reduced frontal activity during a verbal fluency test in fibromyalgia: A near-infrared spectroscopy study.*, *50*, 35-40.

Cope, Z. A. & Young, J. W. J. C. p. i. n. (2017). *The five-choice continuous performance task (5C-CPT): a cross-species relevant paradigm for assessment of vigilance and response inhibition in rodents.*, *78*(1), 9.56. 51-59.56. 18.

Couturier, J., Kimber, M. & Szatmari, P. J. I. J. o. E. D. (2013). *Efficacy of family-based treatment for adolescents with eating disorders: A systematic review and meta-analysis.*, *46*(1), 3-11.

Curtin, M. & Fossey, E. J. A. o. t. j. (2007). *Appraising the trustworthiness of qualitative studies: Guidelines for occupational therapists.*, *54*(2), 88-94.

David, A., Malmberg, A., Lewis, G., Brandt, L. & Allebeck, P. J. S. r. (1995). *Are there neurological and sensory risk factors for schizophrenia?* *14*(3), 247-251.

DeBoskey, D. S. (1982). An investigation of the remediation of learning disabilities based on brain-related tasks as measured by the Halstead-Reitan Neuropsychological Test Battery.

Denes, G. & Pizzamiglio, L. (1999). *Handbook of clinical and experimental neuropsychology*: Psychology Press.

Diamond, G. S., Wintersteen, M. B., Brown, G. K., Diamond, G. M., Gallop, R., Shelef, K. & Psychiatry, A. (2010). *Attachment-based family therapy for adolescents with suicidal ideation: A randomized controlled trial.*, *49*(2), 122-131.

Dickinson, D., Bellack, A. S. & Gold, J. M. J. S. b. (2006). *Social/communication skills, cognition, and vocational functioning in schizophrenia.*, *33*(5), 1213-1220.

Dixon, L., Adams, C. & Lucksted, A. J. S. B. (2000). *Update on family psychoeducation for schizophrenia.*, *26*(1), 5-20.

Donahoe, J. W. (1991). The selectionist approach to verbal behavior: Potential contributions of neuropsychology and connectionism.

Epstein, J. N., Erkanli, A., Conners, C. K., Klaric, J., Costello, J. E. & Angold, A. J. J. o. a. c. p. (2003). *Relations between continuous performance test performance measures and ADHD behaviors.*, *31*(5), 543-554.

Fellows, R. P., Dahmen, J., Cook, D. & Schmitter-Edgecombe, M. J. T. C. N. (2017). *Multicomponent analysis of a digital Trail Making Test.*, *31*(1), 154-167.

Filskov, S. B. & Boll, T. J. (1981). *Handbook of clinical neuropsychology*, (Vol. *1*), Wiley New York.

Fix, J., Rougier, N. & Alexandre, F. J. J. o. P. P. (2007). *From physiological principles to computational models of the cortex.*, *101* (1-3), 32-39.

Fong, T. C., Ho, R. T., Wan, A. H. & Au-Yeung, F. S. J. P. r. (2017). *Psychiatric symptoms mediate the effects of neurological soft signs on functional outcomes in patients with chronic schizophrenia: A longitudinal path-analytic study.*, *249*, 152-158.

Friedlander, M. L., Escudero, V., Heatherington, L. & Diamond, G. M. J. P. (2011). *Alliance in couple and family therapy.*, *48*(1), 25.

Frith, C. D. (2014). *The cognitive neuropsychology of schizophrenia*: Psychology press.

Ghisletta, P., Renaud, O., Fagot, D., Lecerf, T. & De Ribaupierre, A. J. I. J. o. B. D. (2018). *Age and sex differences in intra-individual variability in a simple reaction time task.*, *42*(2), 294-299.

Goghari, V. M., MacDonald III, A. W. & Sponheim, S. R. J. S. b. (2011). *Temporal lobe structures and facial emotion recognition in schizophrenia patients and nonpsychotic relatives.*, *37*(6), 1281-1294.

Goldberg, S., Fruchter, E., Davidson, M., Reichenberg, A., Yoffe, R. & Weiser, M. J. S. b. (2011). *The relationship between risk of hospitalization for schizophrenia, SES, and cognitive functioning.*, *37*(4), 664-670.

Goldstein, S., Naglieri, J. A., Princiotta, D. & Otero, T. M. (2014). Introduction: a history of executive functioning as a theoretical and clinical construct. In *Handbook of executive functioning*, (pp. 3-12), Springer.

Grondhuis, S. N., Mulick, J. A. J. A. J. o. I. & Disabilities, D. (2013). *Comparison of the Leiter International Performance Scale—Revised and the Stanford-Binet Intelligence Scales, in children with autism spectrum disorders.*, *118*(1), 44-54.

Groves, S. J., Porter, R. J., Jordan, J., Knight, R., Carter, J. D., McIntosh, V. V. & Anxiety. (2015). *Changes in neuropsychological function after treatment with metacognitive therapy or cognitive behavior therapy for depression.*, *32*(6), 437-444.

Gur, R. E. J. J. o. a. p. (1978). *Left hemisphere dysfunction and left hemisphere overactivation in schizophrenia.*, *87*(2), 226.

Head, D., Kennedy, K. M., Rodrigue, K. M. & Raz, N. J. N. (2009). *Age differences in perseveration: cognitive and neuroanatomical mediators of performance on the Wisconsin Card Sorting Test.*, *47*(4), 1200-1203.

Heckers, S., Goff, D. & Weiss, A. P. J. P. R. N. (2002). *Reversed hemispheric asymmetry during simple visual perception in schizophrenia.*, *116*(1-2), 25-32.

Heilman, K. M. & Valenstein, E. E. (2003). *Clinical neuropsychology*: Oxford University Press.

Heinssen, R. K., Liberman, R. P. & Kopelowicz, A. J. S. b. (2000). *Psychosocial skills training for schizophrenia: lessons from the laboratory.*, *26*(1), 21-46.

Hewitt, J. & Coffey, M. J. J. o. a. n. (2005). *Therapeutic working relationships with people with schizophrenia: Literature review.*, *52*(5), 561-570.

Higashi, K., Medic, G., Littlewood, K. J., Diez, T., Granström, O. & De Hert, M. J. T. a. i. p. (2013). *Medication adherence in schizophrenia: factors influencing adherence and consequences of nonadherence, a systematic literature review.*, *3*(4), 200-218.

Hofmann, S. G., Asnaani, A., Vonk, I. J., Sawyer, A. T., Fang, A. J. C. t. & research. (2012). *The efficacy of cognitive behavioral therapy: A review of meta-analyses.*, *36*(5), 427-440.

Howes, O., Jauhar, S., Brugger, S. & Pepper, F. J. S. b. (2018). *9.2 brain structural and neurochemical heterogeneity and homogeneity in psychotic disorders: Transdiagnostic PET and MRI imaging findings in schizophrenia and bipolar affective disorder.*, *44*(suppl_1), S13-S13.

Howes, O. D. & Kapur, S. J. S. b. (2009). *The dopamine hypothesis of schizophrenia: version III—the final common pathway.*, *35*(3), 549-562.

Hurford, I. M., Kalkstein, S. & Hurford, M. J. P. T. (2011). *Cognitive rehabilitation in schizophrenia.*, *28*(3), 43-47.

Jasinski, L. J., Berry, D. T., Shandera, A. L., Clark, J. A. J. J. o. C. & Neuropsychology, E. (2011). *Use of the Wechsler Adult Intelligence Scale Digit Span subtest for malingering detection: A meta-analytic review.*, *33*(3), 300-314.

John, S. E. (2016). *The unity and diversity of neuropsychological tasks of executive functioning: Construct and ecological validity of common assessment measures*: University of Colorado at Colorado Springs.

Kaplan, B. J. (2016). Kaplan and Sadock's Synopsis of Psychiatry. Behavioral Sciences/Clinical Psychiatry. *Tijdschrift voor Psychiatrie*, *58*(1), 78-79.

Kaswan, N., Thompson, R., Adler, J. & Hirst, R. J. A. o. C. N. (2019). *A-77 Validity Testing with Youth Populations: D-KEFS Trail Making Test Conditions 4: 2 Ratio as an Embedded Validity Indicator.*, *34*(6), 937-937.

Kaufman, A. S., Flanagan, D. P., Alfonso, V. C. & Mascolo, J. T. J. J. o. P. A. (2006). *Test review: Wechsler intelligence scale for children, (WISC-IV).*, *24*(3), 278-295.

Kent, P. L. (2020). *The Wechsler Memory Scale: A Guide for Clinicians and Researchers*: Routledge.

Kluwe-Schiavon, B., Sanvicente-Vieira, B., Kristensen, C. & Grassi-Oliveira, R. J. J. o. P. R. (2013). *Executive functions rehabilitation for schizophrenia: a critical systematic review.*, *47*(1), 91-104.

Köstering, L., Schmidt, C. S., Egger, K., Amtage, F., Peter, J., Klöppel, S. & Kaller, C. P. J. N. (2015). *Assessment of planning performance in clinical samples: Reliability and validity of the Tower of London task (TOL-F).*, *75*, 646-655.

Krabbendam, L. & Aleman, A. J. P. (2003). *Cognitive rehabilitation in schizophrenia: a quantitative analysis of controlled studies.*, *169*(3-4), 376-382.

Kuhaneck, H. & Watling, R. J. T. A. J. o. O. T. (2015). *Occupational Therapy.*, *69*(5).

Lacro, J. P., Dunn, L. B., Dolder, C. R., Leckband, S. G. & Jeste, D. V. J. T. J. o. c. p. (2002). Prevalence of and risk factors for medication nonadherence in patients with schizophrenia: a comprehensive review of recent literature.

Lambert, M., Bock, T., Schöttle, D., Golks, D., Meister, K., Rietschel, L. & Burlon, M. J. T. J. o. c. p. (2010). Assertive community treatment as part of integrated care versus standard care: a 12-month trial in patients with first-and multiple-episode schizophrenia spectrum disorders treated with quetiapine immediate release (ACCESS trial).

Langeluddecke, P. M. & Lucas, S. K. J. A. o. c. n. (2003). *Quantitative measures of memory malingering on the Wechsler Memory Scale— Third edition in mild head injury litigants. 18*(2), 181-197.

Lauder, S. D., Berk, M., Castle, D. J., Dodd, S. & Berk, L. J. M. j. o. A. (2010). *The role of psychotherapy in bipolar disorder., 193*, S31-S35.

Lebowitz, E. R., Panza, K. E., Su, J. & Bloch, M. H. J. E. R. o. N. (2012). *Family accommodation in obsessive–compulsive disorder., 12*(2), 229-238.

Leucht, S., Corves, C., Arbter, D., Engel, R. R., Li, C. & Davis, J. M. J. T. L. (2009). *Second-generation versus first-generation antipsychotic drugs for schizophrenia: a meta-analysis., 373*(9657), 31-41.

Liberman, R. P. J. S. B. (1986). *Psychiatric rehabilitation of schizophrenia: editor's introduction., 12*(4), 540.

Lieberman, J. A., Stroup, T. S., McEvoy, J. P., Swartz, M. S., Rosenheck, R. A., Perkins, D. O. & Lebowitz, B. D. J. N. E. J. o. M. (2005). *Effectiveness of antipsychotic drugs in patients with chronic schizophrenia., 353*(12), 1209-1223.

Littell, W. M. J. P. B. (1960). *The Wechsler Intelligence Scale for Children: Review of a decade of research., 57*(2), 132.

Lopez, C., Stahl, D. & Tchanturia, K. J. A. o. G. P. (2010). *Estimated intelligence quotient in anorexia nervosa: a systematic review and meta-analysis of the literature., 9*(1), 40.

López, S. B., Borrego, N. S., de la Hera Cabero, M., Carrascal, I. O., Flores, L. & Rico, R. J. J. E. P. (2016). *Neurological symptoms in schizophrenia: A case report., 33*, S573.

Lysaker, P. H., Bell, M. D., Zito, W. S., Bioty, S. M. J. J. o. N. & Disease, M. (1995). Social skills at work: Deficits and predictors of improvement in schizophrenia.

McCrimmon, A. W. & Smith, A. D. (2013). Review of the wechsler abbreviated scale of intelligence, (WASI-II). In: Sage Publications Sage CA: Los Angeles, CA.

McFarlane, W. R., Dixon, L., Lukens, E., Lucksted, A. J. J. o. m. & therapy, f. (2003). *Family psychoeducation and schizophrenia: a review of the literature.*, 29(2), 223-245.

McFarlane, W. R. J. F. P. (2016). *Family interventions for schizophrenia and the psychoses: A review.*, 55(3), 460-482.

Mills, A. & Millsteed, J. J. A. O. T. J. (2002). *Retention: an unresolved workforce issue affecting rural occupational therapy services.*, 49(4), 170-181.

Moray, N. (2017). *Attention: Selective processes in vision and hearing*: Routledge.

Morlett Paredes, A., Carrasco, J., Kamalyan, L., Cherner, M., Umlauf, A., Rivera Mindt, M. & Heaton, R. K. J. T. C. N. (2020). Demographically adjusted normative data for the Halstead category test in a Spanish-speaking adult population: *Results from the Neuropsychological Norms for the US-Mexico Border Region in Spanish (NP-NUMBRS).*, 1-18.

Morris, K., Reid, G. & Spencer, S. J. C. D. o. S. R. (2018). *Occupational therapy delivered by specialists versus non-specialists for people with schizophrenia.*, (10).

Nuechterlein, K. H., Barch, D. M., Gold, J. M., Goldberg, T. E., Green, M. F. & Heaton, R. K. (2004). Identification of separable cognitive factors in schizophrenia. *Schizophrenia Research*, 72(1), 29-39.

O'Halloran, C. J., Kinsella, G. J., Storey, E. J. J. o. c. & neuropsychology, e. (2012). *The cerebellum and neuropsychological functioning: a critical review.*, 34(1), 35-56.

Onitsuka, T., McCarley, R. W., Kuroki, N., Dickey, C. C., Kubicki, M., Demeo, S. S. & Shenton, M. E. J. S. r. (2007). *Occipital lobe gray matter volume in male patients with chronic schizophrenia: A quantitative MRI study.*, 92(1-3), 197-206.

Ono, Y., Kikuchi, M., Nakatani, H., Murakami, M., Nishisaka, M., Muramatsu, T. & Minabe, Y. J. A. j. o. p. (2017). *Prefrontal oxygenation during verbal fluency and cognitive function in adolescents with bipolar disorder type II.*, *25*, 147-153.

Orellana, G. & Slachevsky, A. J. F. i. p. (2013). *Executive functioning in schizophrenia.*, *4*, 35.

Orfanos, S., Banks, C., Priebe, S. J. P. & Psychosomatics. (2015). *Are group psychotherapeutic treatments effective for patients with schizophrenia? A systematic review and meta-analysis.*, *84*(4), 241-249.

Parker, G., Tavella, G., Macqueen, G., Berk, M., Grunze, H., Deckersbach, T. & Malhi, G. S. (2018). Revising Diagnostic and Statistical Manual of Mental Disorders, Fifth Edition, criteria for the bipolar disorders: Phase I of the AREDOC project. *Aust N Z J Psychiatry*, 4867418808382. doi:10.1177/0004867418808382

Pauli-Pott, U. & Becker, K. J. C. P. R. (2011). *Neuropsychological basic deficits in preschoolers at risk for ADHD: A meta-analysis.*, *31*(4), 626-637.

Pekkala, E. T. & Merinder, L. B. J. C. d. o. s. r. (2002). *Psychoeducation for schizophrenia.*, (2).

Pekkonen, E., Katila, H., Ahveninen, J., Karhu, J., Huotilainen, M. & Tiihonen, J. J. S. b. (2002). *Impaired temporal lobe processing of preattentive auditory discrimination in schizophrenia.*, *28*(3), 467-474.

Phillips, L. H. J. M. (1999). *The role of memory in the Tower of London task.*, *7*(2), 209-231.

Picchioni, M. M., Rijsdijk, F., Toulopoulou, T., Chaddock, C., Cole, J. H., Ettinger, U. & JPN, n. (2017). *Familial and environmental influences on brain volumes in twins with schizophrenia.*, *42*(2), 122.

Porter, R. J., Bourke, C., Gallagher, P. J. A. & Psychiatry, N. Z. J. o. (2007). *Neuropsychological impairment in major depression: its nature, origin and clinical significance.*, *41*(2), 115-128.

Randolph, J. J. J. A. N. A. (2018). *Positive neuropsychology: The science and practice of promoting cognitive health.*, *25*(4), 287-294.

Rapport, M. D., Orban, S. A., Kofler, M. J. & Friedman, L. M. J. C. p. r. (2013). Do programs designed to train working memory, other executive functions, and attention benefit children with ADHD? *A meta-analytic review of cognitive, academic, and behavioral outcomes.*, *33*(8), 1237-1252.

Rhodes, M. G. J. P. & aging. (2004). *Age-related differences in performance on the Wisconsin card sorting test: a meta-analytic review.*, *19*(3), 482.

Roid, G. H. & Pomplun, M. (2012). *The stanford-binet intelligence scales*: The Guilford Press.

Rowe, C. L. J. J. o. m. & therapy, f. (2012). *Family therapy for drug abuse: Review and updates 2003–2010.*, *38*(1), 59-81.

Rummel-Kluge, C., Komossa, K., Schwarz, S., Hunger, H., Schmid, F., Lobos, C. A. & Leucht, S. J. S. r. (2010). *Head-to-head comparisons of metabolic side effects of second generation antipsychotics in the treatment of schizophrenia: a systematic review and meta-analysis.*, *123*(2-3), 225-233.

Sapara, A., Cooke, M., Fannon, D., Francis, A., Buchanan, R. W., Anilkumar, A. P. & Kumari, V. J. S. r. (2007). *Prefrontal cortex and insight in schizophrenia: a volumetric MRI study.*, *89*(1-3), 22-34.

Sarin, F., Wallin, L. & Widerlöv, B. J. N. j. o. p. (2011). *Cognitive behavior therapy for schizophrenia: a meta-analytical review of randomized controlled trials.*, *65*(3), 162-174.

Schaefer, M., Sarkar, S., Theophil, I., Leopold, K., Heinz, A. & Gallinat, J. J. P. (2019). Acute and Long-term Memantine Add-on Treatment to Risperidone Improves Cognitive Dysfunction in Patients with Acute and Chronic Schizophrenia.

Schneider, H. E., Lam, J. C. & Mahone, E. M. J. C. N. (2016). *Sleep disturbance and neuropsychological function in young children with ADHD.*, *22*(4), 493-506.

Schneider, S., Blatter-Meunier, J., Herren, C., In-Albon, T., Adornetto, C., Meyer, A. & psychology, c. (2013). *The efficacy of a family-based cognitive-behavioral treatment for separation anxiety disorder in children aged 8–13: A randomized comparison with a general anxiety program.*, *81*(5), 932.

Schoenberg, M. R. & Scott, J. G. (2011). *The little black book of neuropsychology: a syndrome-based approach*: Springer.

Shallice, T. (1988). *From neuropsychology to mental structure*: Cambridge University Press.

Smerud, P. E. & Rosenfarb, I. S. (2011). *The therapeutic alliance and family psychoeducation in the treatment of schizophrenia: An exploratory prospective change process study.*

Sporns, O. J. D. i. c. n. (2013). *Structure and function of complex brain networks.*, *15*(3), 247.

Spreen, O., Risser, A. H. & Edgell, D. (1995). *Developmental neuropsychology*: Oxford University Press, USA.

Stahl, S. M. J. C. s. (2018). *Beyond the dopamine hypothesis of schizophrenia to three neural networks of psychosis: dopamine, serotonin, and glutamate.*, *23*(3), 187-191.

Stapleton, T. & McBrearty, C. J. B. J. o. O. T. (2009). *Use of standardised assessments and outcome measures among a sample of Irish occupational therapists working with adults with physical disabilities.*, *72*(2), 55-64.

Suddath, R. L., Christison, G. W., Torrey, E. F., Casanova, M. F. & Weinberger, D. R. J. N. E. J. o. M. (1990). *Anatomical abnormalities in the brains of monozygotic twins discordant for schizophrenia.*, *322*(12), 789-794.

Summers, M. J. & Saunders, N. L. J. N. (2012). *Neuropsychological measures predict decline to Alzheimer's dementia from mild cognitive impairment.*, *26*(4), 498.

Tchanturia, K., Davies, H., Roberts, M., Harrison, A., Nakazato, M., Schmidt, U. & Morris, R. J. P. o. (2012). *Poor cognitive flexibility in eating disorders: examining the evidence using the Wisconsin Card Sorting Task.*, *7*(1).

Teive, H. A., Teive, G. M., Dallabrida, N. & Gutierrez, L. J. A. d. n. p. (2017). *Alfred Binet: Charcot's pupil, a neuropsychologist and a pioneer in intelligence testing.*, *75*(9), 673-675.

Thieda, P., Beard, S., Richter, A. & Kane, J. J. P. s. (2003). *An economic review of compliance with medication therapy in the treatment of schizophrenia.*, *54*(4), 508-516.

Tohid, H., Faizan, M. & Faizan, U. J. N. (2015). *Alterations of the occipital lobe in schizophrenia.*, *20*(3), 213.

Torrey, E. F. J. S. r. (2007). *Schizophrenia and the inferior parietal lobule.*, *97*(1-3), 215-225.

Van Den Heuvel, O. A., Groenewegen, H. J., Barkhof, F., Lazeron, R. H., Van Dyck, R. & Veltman, D. J. J. N. (2003). *Frontostriatal system in planning complexity: a parametric functional magnetic resonance version of Tower of London task.*, *18*(2), 367-374.

van Haren, N. J. J. o. t. A. A. o. C. & Psychiatry, A. (2017). *8.1 Brain Abnormalities and IQ in Offspring Related to Those in Siblings, Co-Twins, and Parents of Patients With Schizophrenia.*, *56*(10), S313.

Vancampfort, D., De Hert, M., Skjerven, L. H., Gyllensten, A. L., Parker, A., Mulders, N. & rehabilitation. (2012). *International Organization of Physical Therapy in Mental Health consensus on physical activity within multidisciplinary rehabilitation programmes for minimising cardio-metabolic risk in patients with schizophrenia.*, *34*(1), 1-12.

Walsh, K. W. (1978). *Neuropsychology: A clinical approach*: Churchill Livingstone.

Watkins, M. W. J. P. a. (2006). *Orthogonal higher order structure of the Wechsler Intelligence Scale for Children.*, *18*(1), 123.

Wechsler, D. J. T. P. C. S. A. & TX. (2012). Wechsler preschool and primary scale of intelligence—fourth edition.

Weintraub, S., Wicklund, A. H. & Salmon, D. P. J. C. S. H. p. i. m. (2012). *The neuropsychological profile of Alzheimer disease.*, *2*(4), a006171.

Willoughby, M., Hong, Y., Hudson, K. & Wylie, A. J. J. o. E. C. P. (2020). *Between-and within-person contributions of simple reaction time to executive function skills in early childhood.*, *104779*.

Wing, V. C., Moss, T. G., Rabin, R. A. & George, T. P. J. A. B. (2012). *Effects of cigarette smoking status on delay discounting in schizophrenia and healthy controls.*, *37*(1), 67-72.

Wingard, E., Barrett, A., Crucian, G., Doty, L., Heilman, K. J. J. o. N. & Neurosurgery & Psychiatry. (2002). *The Gerstmann syndrome in Alzheimer's disease.*, *72*(3), 403-405.

Wong, B. (2011). *Learning about learning disabilities*: Elsevier.

Ye, F., Zhan, Q., Xiao, W., Sha, W. & Zhang, X. J. I. j. o. m. i. p. r. (2018). *Altered serum levels of glial cell line-derived neurotrophic factor in male chronic schizophrenia patients with tardive dyskinesia.*, *27*(4), e1727.

Zervas, I. M., Theleritis, C. & Soldatos, C. R. J. T. W. J. o. B. P. (2012). *Using ECT in schizophrenia: a review from a clinical perspective.*, *13*(2), 96-105.

Zhou, S. Y., Suzuki, M., Takahashi, T., Hagino, H., Kawasaki, Y., Matsui, M. & Kurachi, M. J. S. r. (2007). *Parietal lobe volume deficits in schizophrenia spectrum disorders.*, *89*(1-3), 35-48.

In: Schizophrenia
Editor: Bojan Sterenborg
ISBN: 978-1-53618-144-9
© 2020 Nova Science Publishers, Inc.

Chapter 2

BLOOD BIOMARKERS IN SCHIZOPHRENIA: A FOCUS ON GENETICS

Javier Gilabert-Juan[1,*], *PhD*
and Andrzej W. Cwetsch[2,3], *PhD*

[1]Center for Interdisciplinary Research in Biology, College de France, Paris, France
[2]Institut de Psychiatrie et Neuroscience de Paris, INSERM, Paris, France
[3]Imagine - Institut des maladies génétiques, Paris, France

ABSTRACT

Schizophrenia is a chronic mental disorder characterized by abnormal behavior and a decreased ability to interpret reality. Due to its complexity, during the last few years, many efforts have been made to understand the etiology of the disease and to describe the genetic background responsible for its development. Indeed, numerous studies associated several genes and genetic variants to the pathology. Nevertheless, classical gene studies could not characterize a genetic pool that identifies a specific profile of the patients with schizophrenia. Thus, it is necessary to find genetic expression patterns that allow us to delimit

---

* Corresponding Author's E-mail: javier.gilabert@college-de-france.fr.

different phenotypes of the disease. Genetic variations and markers can serve as a diagnostic, prognostic and therapeutic tool for the patients. However, limited access to the brain led researchers to look for other, easier to obtain, tissue for marker identification such as peripheral blood. Indeed, many investigations have shown that gene expression in the brain is blood-correlated. Interestingly, genetic markers found in blood include epigenetic changes, alterations in the gene expression and miRNA identification. Here, we describe and summarize the blood-based biomarkers of schizophrenia from the diagnostic, prognostic and therapeutic point of view. Finally, we will further discuss the future perspectives and the translational aspect of the latest discoveries in the field of schizophrenia research.

1. INTRODUCTION

Schizophrenia is a mental disease affecting 1% of the total population worldwide (Moreno-Küstner, Martín, and Pastor 2018). Despite the large number of individuals affected by this disease, we still do not know the exact genetic and environmental causes of the condition. Indeed, over the last few years, multiple genes have been associated with the disease presenting different weights and characteristics associated with schizophrenia symptoms. A growing list of genetic polymorphisms, rare genetic variants, *de novo* mutations, epigenetic changes and other genomic alterations showing a connection with schizophrenia have been provided. However, despite that numerous genes are linked to the disease, there is currently no clinical test that can offer diagnostic or prognostic utility. Thus, it is important to know the markers of the disease, at different levels, that can, from a clinical point of view, help classify patients in the early onset of symptoms.

Genetic markers or gene expression markers are an interesting source of information in many pathological conditions. Regarding the gene expression studies in postmortem brain tissues, genetic heterogeneity in schizophrenia has been revealed. Furthermore, the involvement of different biological pathways appeared as a possible susceptibility factor of the disease. As a consequence, in the last few years, a huge effort has been made in the field of schizophrenia to detect the specific causes of the particular symptoms of the disease, promoting studies in endophenotypes (also known as intermediate phenotypes). Nevertheless, since a brain biopsy is a very invasive procedure, the translation of this knowledge into the clinics as a diagnostic tool seems to be far from perfect. At this point, more accessible tissue should be used in order to obtain reliable and indicative material for gene-expression alteration studies in patients with schizophrenia.

One of the most accessible human tissue is the blood. Indeed, blood samples are widely used for disease assessment because of the low invasiveness of the sampling procedure. Moreover, because blood cells are in contact with tissue throughout the body, gene expression in blood mirrors the gene expression in other organs. The identification of blood biomarkers for schizophrenia risk assessment has become a new and promising area of translational investigation in psychiatry. Biomarkers identified from gene expression studies may better reflect the complex etiology of schizophrenia, since environmental triggers can influence gene transcription levels. Furthermore, a large number of studies have indicated that alterations in central nervous system genes may affect metabolism and gene expression in the peripheral blood through neurotransmitters, cytokines or hormones. Finally, peripheral blood biomarkers may also be useful as indicators of endophenotypes. Thus, a precise description of different subtypes of patients identified by characteristics such as the age of onset or the response to the treatment associated with blood-markers for these endophenotypes, will help in a better prognosis and specialized therapeutics in the future.

In this chapter we are going to summarize and comment on some of the most interesting studies performed in the field of biomarker research in peripheral blood of patients with schizophrenia. Moreover, we will describe some of the work that has attempted to offer diagnostic, prognostic or therapeutic value. We will also indicate the possible benefits, as well as weaknesses, of certain biomarkers as candidates for a schizophrenia diagnosis. Finally, we will classify the different studies regarding the type of markers and the pathways studied.

1.1. Neurotransmitters

The dopamine and serotonin systems have largely been associated to schizophrenia in several studies. This is mainly due to the fact that antipsychotic drugs such as clozapine, olanzapine, quetiapine, risperidone, and ziprasidone among others are potent serotonin and dopamine receptor antagonists (Meltzer 1999). One of the first studies in dopaminergic markers of schizophrenia in blood used quantitative Polymerase Chain Reaction (qPCR) to show that *dopamine receptor D3* mRNA is increased in patients with schizophrenia at least 2-fold compared to healthy controls without significant alterations in the mRNA of the *D4 receptor* (Vogel et al. 2004). This increase in *D3 receptor* expression is not affected by different antipsychotic drug treatments. In addition, drug-naïve patients exhibit the same increase in mRNA expression, indicating that this change is not a result of medical treatment (Ilani 2001). The main caveat of this study is the very low number of patients and controls, 14 and 11 respectively. The same year, another study in 44 medicated patients with schizophrenia (followed for more than 3 years), 28 unmedicated patients (followed for more than 3 months), 15 drug-naïve patients and 31 healthy controls indicated (by qPCR) that in unmedicated patients, the *D3 dopamine receptor* mRNA of peripheral lymphocytes was significantly increased compared to that of healthy controls and medicated patients. The study showed as well that the *D5 dopamine receptor* mRNA level was increased compared to that of medicated patients with schizophrenia (Kwak et al. 2001). Interestingly, after two weeks of medication, the mRNA of dopamine receptors peaked, followed by a decrease during subsequent weeks. When unmedicated and drug-naïve patients were divided into two groups according to dopamine receptor expression before medication, they observed that the group with increased expression of the dopamine receptors showed more severe psychiatric symptoms (Kwak et al. 2001). In 2006, the expression of *D3* and *D4 dopamine receptors* was studied in neutrophils, monocytes, B cells, natural killer cells and $CD4^+$- and $CD8^+$-T lymphocytes by qPCR (Boneberg et al. 2006). An increased expression of *D3 receptor* mRNA in T cells of schizophrenic patients was found, whereas *D4* mRNA in $CD4^+$-T cells was downregulated (Boneberg et al. 2006). Nevertheless, this study was performed in 10 patients compared to 10 healthy controls. In contrast to the previous studies, Vogel et al., in 2004 showed a decreased amount of *D3* mRNA in the blood of patients with schizophrenia when compared to healthy controls. Interestingly, after the treatment with antipsychotics, *D3* levels reached similar values as those of healthy controls. Thus, this can support the hypothesis of altered neurotransmitter system in schizophrenia disease, and more specific studies considering the endophenotype of the patients should be carried out to determine in which cases *D3* can be used as a marker of the disease status (Vogel et al. 2004).

Regarding *D2 dopamine receptor*, an increase of the mRNA of this receptor has also been observed in blood of patients with schizophrenia. The *D2 receptor* and the *inwardly rectifying potassium channel gene (Kir2.3)* were found to be increased in a microarray study involving 13 patients (Zvara et al. 2005). Subsequently, this was also confirmed by qPCR. Interestingly, in a more recent study performed in 25 acute patients with schizophrenia, 27 chronic patients and 30 healthy controls, the *D2 receptor* mRNA levels did not differ between the three groups but correlated with positive symptoms in acute patients. In contrast, dopamine transporter mRNA levels were higher in chronic patients compared to healthy controls. In this case, the *D2 receptor* would not be a good marker of the disease but possibly a good indicator of the early onset of the disease and the acute symptoms (Zvara et al. 2005).

An interesting endophenotype in schizophrenia is the existence of treatment-resistant patients. This specific group of patients are the ones that do not respond to the drug treatment independent of the time suffering from the disease. Thus, we can find treatment-resistant patients after the first episode of psychosis or in chronic disease cases. In this context, it is very important to find biological markers that could predict the response to antipsychotic drugs and, consequently, improve the prognosis of the patients. In 2018 a study carried out by Moretti et al. failed to find any gene expression biomarker in the blood of 78 treatment-resistant patients with schizophrenia (Moretti et al. 2018). This group compared the expression profile of several genes previously associated with schizophrenia (*COMT, CNR1, TNF, DISC1, PAFAH1B1, NDEL1, MBP, AKT1, DGCR8, DICER1, DROSHA, UFD1L* and *DGCR2*). Despite the lack of association with the response to the treatment, they found two genes related to the disease pathophysiology: the *cannabinoid receptor 1* (*CNR1*) and the *Ubiquitin Recognition Factor In ER Associated Degradation 1* (*UFD1L*), that were differentially expressed in the blood of patients with schizophrenia when compared to healthy controls (Moretti et al. 2018).

1.2. Immune System

One of the proposed systems involved in the etiology of schizophrenia is the immune system. Indeed, chronically-activated macrophages and T cells have been observed in patients suffering from schizophrenia and other psychiatric disorders (Smith 1992). Several studies showed a proinflammatory profile in the brain as well as in blood samples of schizophrenic patients (Upthegrove, Manzanares-Teson, and Barnes 2014; Hess et al. 2016). Some of these studies suggest that the activation of the immune system could accompany the acute phase of the psychosis (Smith and Maes 1995). Confirming this hypothesis, a recent study focused on acute phase proteins (APP) showed that the mRNA of the *haptoglobin* (*HP*) gene was increased in patients during the first recruitment and after one and three months from the disease onset (Yee et al. 2017). Furthermore, they showed that antitrypsin (A1T) gene expression was significantly higher in controls compared to patients at the 1-month follow-up visit. Finally, the patients had significantly higher *alpha-2 macroglobulin* (*A2M*) gene expression than controls at the 3-month follow-up visit (Yee et al. 2017).

Transforming growth factor beta 1 (*TGF-β1*) is a member of the growth factor beta family of cytokines, which inhibits the production of Th1 cytokines including interferon-g (IFN-γ), tumor necrosis factor-α (TNFα), IL2, and IL2R (Grayson et al. 2006; Gibb et al. 2008; Gallego et al. 2018). In a study of 15 medication-free patients and 15 healthy controls, the level of mRNAs including *TGF-β1, IL-1β, IL-23, TNFα, NF-κB,* and *BDNF* were analyzed (Amoli et al. 2019). *TGF-β1* was significantly up-regulated in peripheral blood of patients with schizophrenia compared to healthy controls. In addition, the same study found a significant correlation between the positive symptom scale and *TGF-β1* gene expression (Amoli et al. 2019). Despite the low sample numbers, these results are interesting since they show possible markers in unmedicated patients and therefore not influenced by the effect of antipsychotics.

Tumor Necrosis Factor (TNF) is one of the proinflammatory cytokines. It is expressed by neurons, astrocytes, some microglia cells and endothelial cells (Aggarwal 2003). *TNF* is recognized mainly by two membrane-bound receptors: the *TNF receptor 1 (TNFR1)* and *TNF receptor 2 (TNFR2)*, which are distributed in a range of cells including immune cells, endothelial cells, specific neuronal subtypes and glia cells (Tecchio, Micheletti, and Cassatella 2014). In 2010, using semiquantitative methods, Liu and colleges showed that the mRNA expression levels of *TNF-α* in peripheral blood were significantly increased in patients with schizophrenia (3-fold) as compared with healthy control subjects and positively correlated with the Positive And Negative Schizophrenia Symptoms (PANSS), a general psychopathology subscale score of these patients (L. Liu et al. 2010). The results of this study were supported by one of Drexhage et al., 2010 which, through Taqman probes, showed an increase of the mRNA of *TNF-α* gene in the blood of patients with schizophrenia (Drexhage et al. 2010). A recent paper showed that TNF protein is also slightly increased in the plasma of schizophrenic patients compared to healthy controls (Hoseth et al. 2017). Moreover, the two TNF receptors were increased in the blood of these patients suggesting a subtle but potentially biologically relevant proinflammatory imbalance in the TNF system of patients with schizophrenia (Hoseth et al. 2017). Nevertheless, when they address the alterations of these molecules at the mRNA level, they observed a decrease of *TNF-α* mRNA suggesting other cellular sources of plasmatic *TNF-α* than circulating leukocytes and eliminating *TNF-α* mRNA as a good candidate for schizophrenic markers in blood (Hoseth et al. 2017).

The cannabinoid system exerts regulatory functions in both immune and central nervous systems. Some of the controlled functions of the cannabinoid system are those related closely to schizophrenic symptoms such as emotional processing and cognition (DeRosse et al. 2010; Rabin, Zakzanis, and George 2011). Interestingly, in the peripheral mononuclear blood cells, the cannabinoid receptors *CB1R* and *CB2R* are shown to either increase or suppress T-cell and B-cell functions which closely links this system with the immune system (Suárez-Pinilla et al. 2015). Indeed, *CB1R* and *CB2R* mRNAs were slightly increased in the blood of patients with schizophrenia when compared to healthy controls and positively correlated with PANSS, which makes these two genes good candidates as biomarkers of a general disease status (Chase et al. 2016).

In a recent paper, Ukkola Vuoti et al., studied markers of cognitive endophenotypes in 74 patients with schizophrenia (Ukkola-Vuoti et al. 2019). With a genome-wide gene expression chip, they showed that the most significant genetic associations were: *Reticulon 4* (*RTN4*), a gene associated with an endophenotype factor of Processing Speed in patients, *Family with Sequence Similarity 89 Member A* (*FAM89A*), a gene related to Verbal Working Memory, and *HYDIN Axonemal Central Pair Apparatus Protein* (*HYDIN*) which is associated with Recognition Memory (Ukkola-Vuoti et al. 2019). When the pathway analysis was performed, the genes associated with cognitive endophenotypes were enriched for functions in immune or inflammatory mechanisms, including EIF2 signaling, antigen presentation, as well as in molecular and cellular functions related to cell death and survival (Ukkola-Vuoti et al. 2019). In the same line, the study of Gilabert-Juan et al., 2019 in two different cohorts showed, primarily by qPCR, increased expression of the *Eukaryotic Translation Initiation Factor 2D* (*EIF2D*) and *Thymocyte Selection-Associated High Mobility Group Box* (*TOX*) genes in a chronic patient group compared to healthy controls (Gilabert-Juan et al. 2019). *EIF2D* encodes a factor involved in a non-canonical translation initiation mechanism of protein synthesis that is believed to operate mainly in cells under stress, and *TOX* is an evolutionarily conserved member of the HMG-box family of transcription factors that has been mainly studied in the immune system (Dmitriev et al. 2010; Aliahmad, De La Torre, and Kaye 2010). Despite these results, in the second cohort of patients with acute psychotic phenotype, *EIF2D* was significantly reduced and *TOX* did not showed differences between patient and control groups. Accordingly, a study by Gardiner et al., 2013 by microarray technique in 114 patients with schizophrenia and 80 healthy controls showed altered expression of several genes involved mostly in immunological response pathway (E. J. Gardiner et al. 2013). Only six genes were confirmed altered by qPCR: *EIF2C2* (*Ago 2*), *MEF2D*, *EVL*, *PI3*, *S100A12* and *DEFA4* (E. J. Gardiner et al. 2013). These three studies point out the interest of the *EIF2* signaling pathway for understanding the etiology of the disease and for the use of blood biomarkers at different stages of the disease and for cognitive phenotypes.

Toll-like receptors (TLRs) are a family of cellular receptors playing a crucial role in the activation of innate immunity (Kozłowska et al. 2019). A recent study carried out by Kozłowska and coworkers in 27 patients with schizophrenia and 29 healthy controls showed that from the nine Toll-like receptors analyzed by qPCR, the mRNA expression levels of *TLR1, TLR2, TLR4, TLR6*, and *TLR9* were downregulated in patients, whereas those of *TLR3* and *TLR7* were up-regulated (Kozłowska et al. 2019). No differences in *TLR5* and *TLR8* expression were observed between patients and controls (Kozłowska et al. 2019). These results are interesting and open a new possible option for schizophrenia markers in blood; nevertheless, the low number of samples should be taken into consideration and a replication study in a bigger sample should confirm the dysregulation in this family of receptors.

1.3. Hormones

Schizophrenia is a disease affecting twice as many men than women. This fact strengthens the possibility that hormonal regulation is involved in the etiology of the disease (Heringa et al. 2015). Ghrelin is an appetite hormone originally identified in the rodent stomach and plays an important role in sleep regulation, mood, reward, and cognition (Kojima et al. 1999;

Kluge et al. 2008; Chuang and Zigman 2010; Jerlhag et al. 2009; Andrews 2011). A recent study on a Japanese population of 49 patients with schizophrenia and 50 healthy controls interrogates the expression of different genes involved on the Ghrelin signaling pathway (Nakata et al. 2019). They found that mRNA levels of *growth hormone secretagogue receptor 1a* (*GHSR1a*) were lower in patients with schizophrenia than in controls (Nakata et al. 2019). However, *growth hormone secretagogue receptor 1b* (*GHSR1b*) and *membrane bound O-acyltransferase 4* (*MBOAT4*) mRNA expression levels were higher in patients (Nakata et al. 2019). These findings suggest that lower *GHS-R1a* and elevated *GHS-R1b* and *MBOAT4* mRNA expression levels may reflect attenuation of the neuroprotective effects of ghrelin in the patients and can also be used as markers of the disease.

Long non-coding RNAs (lncRNAs) are RNAs involved in regulation of the transcription. These lncRNAs execute this function by binding to histone-modifying proteins, transcription factors and RNA polymerase II (Long et al. 2017). A recent study evaluating different lncRNAs involved in brain development or function regulation, performed in 60 patients with schizophrenia and 60 healthy controls, has shown that RNA from *HOXA-AS2, Linc-ROR, MEG3, SPRY4-IT1* and *UCA1* genes is significantly increased in patients with schizophrenia when compared to healthy controls (Fallah et al. 2019). Nevertheless, this significance was only achieved among females, which makes these genes candidates for sex-specific markers of the disease, and possible genes influenced by hormonal regulations.

1.4. Developmental Genes

The search for good markers in first episode patients with schizophrenia is of critical importance since these patients can be un- or marginally-medicated. Such markers can serve as a diagnostic tool but also can decipher the systems and pathways that are found altered during the development of the disease. A study carried out in 53 first-episode patients with schizophrenia and 73 healthy controls analyzed several genes involved in the disease phenotype (*COMT, TNF, DISC1, PAFAH1B1, NDEL1, MBP, AKT1, DGCR8, DICER1, DROSHA, UFD1L* and *DGCR2*) (Ota et al. 2019; 2015). Interestingly, using qPCR, they identified two genes, the *myelin basic protein* and *nuclear distribution protein nudE-like 1* (*MBP* and *NDEL1*) exhibiting higher expression levels in antipsychotic-naïve first-episode patients than in healthy controls, suggesting potential diagnostic specificities (Ota et al. 2015). MBP is a protein participating in the process of nerve myelination while *NDEL1* encodes a thiol-activated oligopeptidase, playing a role in nervous system development. Both genes have been previously associated to schizophrenic phenotype in early stages of the disease (Yu et al. 2014; Ota et al. 2015).

1.5. Cell Cycle

Cell cycle-related genes have also been studied as biomarkers in schizophrenia even though they have not classically been associated with the disease or with mood disorders. Nevertheless, it is well established that genomic mutations likely occur during chromosomal DNA replication in the cell cycle, and schizophrenia disease is widely associated to these genomic alterations, suggesting that perturbation of the cell cycle may be associated with the disease (Koren et al. 2012). In 2016, Okazaki and colleagues studied 43 genes related to cell-cycle proteins with qPCR, first in a discovery sample (40 patients and 20 healthy controls), then in a replication sample (82 patients and 74 healthy controls) and finally in an intervention group (22 patients and 18 healthy controls) (Okazaki et al. 2016). The sample showed significant differences in the expression of 13 genes: *CDK10, CDK4, CHEK2, MCM3, MCM4, MCM5, MCM6, MCM7, MCM8, ORC3L, POLB, POLD2* and *POLD4*. After, the replication sample confirmed nine genes were expressed significantly differently between the groups: *CDK10, CDK4, MCM3, MCM4, MCM5, MCM6, MCM7, POLD2* and *POLD4* (Okazaki et al. 2016). With these nine genes, a multivariate logistic regression analysis was performed to determine whether mRNA expression levels could be used as biomarkers for schizophrenia, identifying a combination of three genes: *Cyclin-dependent kinase 4* (*CDK4*), *DNA replication licensing factor MCM7* (*MCM7*) and *DNA Polymerase Delta 4* (*POLD4*) as potential candidates (Okazaki et al. 2016). CDK4 is part of a protein kinase complex which is involved in controlling progression through the G1 phase, MCM7 is an essential component for the initiation of genome replication and POLD4 plays a critical role in DNA replication and repair. mRNA expression levels of *CDK4*, *MCM7* and *POLD4* were measured in the intervention group, and in acute patients' samples. The expression of *CDK4* and *MCM7* was significantly decreased in acute state patients, while the expression of *POLD4* was significantly decreased both in acute patients and in patients in remission (Okazaki et al. 2016). In addition, the decreased expression of *CDK4* in acute patients was significantly recovered in remitted patients. These results show that genes related to cell cycle activities can be good markers for the schizophrenic phenotype, but better studies are necessary in order to better associate the acute, chronic and remitted phenotypes to these markers.

RAC-alpha serine/threonine-protein kinase (*AKT1*) is an oncogene implicated in the regulation of the cell cycle (Staal 1987). This gene expression was found to be altered in 10 drug-naïve patients with schizophrenia compared to 10 healthy controls (Kumarasinghe et al. 2013). The levels of *AKT1* went back to normal after eight weeks of treatment, indicating that this gene and its pathway are good potential markers for unmedicated schizophrenic patients (Kumarasinghe et al. 2013). Another study in 12 drug-naïve patients showed alterations in immune response pathways and cell cycle control (Mas et al. 2015). In contrast, in a different study, there was a decrease in *AKT1* mRNA in the blood of drug-naive patients (N=11), in psychotic patients (N=20) and in remitted patients (N=21) when compared to healthy controls (van Beveren et al. 2012). Nevertheless, more studies with a bigger sample size are necessary to confirm these results and to unravel the role of *AKT1* in the etiology of the disease and potentially as biomarker.

1.6. Mitochondrial Metabolism

Accumulating data over the last few years highlights the involvement of mitochondria metabolism in psychiatric disorders since the brain has the highest mitochondrial energy demand of any organ (Pei and Wallace 2018). A recent study using peripheral blood from 131 first episode patients of psychosis and 149 healthy controls showed that 978 genes were differentially expressed between the two groups, through an RNA microarray, and there was an enriched pathway associated with immune function and mitochondrial metabolism (Leirer et al. 2019). But the involvement of the mitochondrial genes as markers of schizophrenia is not only a current point of interest.

A study in 2006 observed that mitochondrial mRNA of the *NADH: Ubiquinone Oxidoreductase Core Subunit S1* (*NDUFS1* or *complex I 75-KDa subunit*) was increased in the blood of 10 first-episode, drug-naïve patients with schizophrenia compared to 10 healthy controls (Mehler-Wex et al. 2006). Three years later, a bigger screening including 12 new patients with schizophrenia at the moment of their first episode was carried out (Taurines et al. 2010). This study confirmed the increased mRNA of the mitochondrial *NDUFS1* in the blood of first episode patients. Nevertheless, the mitochondrial complex I is composed of 44 genes, that have been already classified as biomarkers of the schizophrenia disease (Taurines et al. 2010). More recent studies showed a marked dysregulation in the expression of complex I genes in patients with schizophrenia compared to healthy controls (Haghighatfard et al. 2018). The mRNA levels of different genes associated to the mitochondrial complex 1 were studied by qPCR in 634 patients compared to 528 healthy controls. *NDUFS1, NDUFS4, NDUFV1, NDUFV2, NDUFB2, NDUFB5, NDUFB9, NDUFA5, NDUFA8, NDUFA13* and *NDUFC1* mRNA levels were found increased in patients, while levels of *NDUFAB1, NDUFB10, NDUFB11, NDUFA1, NDUFA2, NDUFS7* and *NDUFS8* were decreased (Haghighatfard et al. 2018). Thus, *NDUFS1* is a possible marker for schizophrenia disease and supports the theory of dysregulation of the respiratory system and mitochondrial metabolism in patients suffering from psychiatric disorders.

1.7. Microarray studies

Microarray provides a basis to genotype thousands of different loci at the same time. It is a useful tool for association and linkage studies to isolate chromosomal regions related to a particular disease. In fact, Bowden et al. 2006 performed a microarray study with 14 patients with schizophrenia and 14 healthy controls, pointing out that 18 genes with brain-related functions were altered (Bowden et al. 2006). From this pool of genes, four were confirmed altered, according to qPCR: *endothelial differentiation gene 2* (*Edg-2*), *ezrin–radixin–moesin phosphoprotein 50* (*EBP50*), *Myc-associated zinc finger protein* (*MAZ*) and *Tumor Necrosis Factor Receptor 2* (*TNFR2*) (Bowden et al. 2006). Another microarray expression study in 32 first episode unmedicated patients compared to 32 healthy controls observed that the actin assembly factor *Dishevelled Associated Activator of Morphogenesis 2* (*DAAM2*) was increased in the patients' samples, and it was confirmed by qPCR (Kuzman et al. 2009). Surprisingly, *DAAM2* mRNA levels returned to control levels in the patients who achieved total clinical remission after nine weeks of treatment. These results suggest that *DAAM2* could be used as a biomarker of disease progression or response to treatment (Kuzman et al. 2009). Interestingly, *DAAM2* is expressed in brain tissue where neuronal differentiation is regulated and it has previously been associated to schizophrenia susceptibility in a Chinese population (Kida, Shiraishi, and Ogura 2004; Proitsi et al. 2008).

Takahashi et al, in 2010 performed a gene expression study in blood of 52 patients with schizophrenia and 49 healthy controls to identify markers of the disease that can be also expressed in the brain (Takahashi et al. 2010). They found 14 altered genes in the blood samples of the patients that could be used as a diagnostic tool. Some of the identified genes are *cyclin-dependent kinase 2-integrating protein* (*CINP*), *Tudor domain containing 9* (*TDRD9*), *d-amino acid oxidase activator* (*DAOA-G72*), *progesterone receptor membrane component 1* (*PGRMC1*), *nuclear assembly factor 1 homolog* (*NAF1*), *lipaze member H* (*LIPH*), *methionine aminopeptidase 1D* (*MAP1D*) and *insulin-like 3* (*INSL3*)(Takahashi et al. 2010). The predictive model they developed reached up to 87.9% accuracy with 82.4% sensitivity and 93.8% specificity in the studied sample (Takahashi et al. 2010).

Comparing genetic profiles of schizophrenic patients with their healthy first-degree biological relatives can give us information about the altered routes that can influence the development of the disease. A study comparing the genetic expression profile in the blood of nine schizophrenic patients with their siblings (N=9) and healthy controls (N=12) pointed out genes involved in nucleosome and histone structure and function in both patients and relatives, suggesting a potential epigenetic mechanism underlying the risk state for the disorder (Glatt et al. 2011).

1.8. MicroRNAs

MicroRNAs (miRNAs) are a class of endogenous small non-coding RNAs that function as post-transcriptional regulators of gene expression. The standard length is about 22 nucleotides and many of them present evolutionarily conserved sequences. The first miRNA was discovered in *Caenorhabditis elegans* in 1993 (Lee, Feinbaum, and Ambros 1993). Since that moment, extensive studies have helped identify thousands of miRNA in various species of animals, plants, and viruses. Indeed, in mammals, especially in the central nervous system, miRNA expression is developmentally regulated and correlates with cortical maturation, including neurite outgrowth, dendritogenesis and dendritic spine formation (Cho et al. 2019). The importance of miRNA in the mammalian brain can also be underlined by the fact that 70% of the known miRNAs are expressed in the mammalian brain (Fineberg, Kosik, and Davidson 2009). Interestingly, genes encoding miRNAs or components in the miRNA biogenesis machinery have been implicated in psychiatric disorders such as schizophrenia (Beveridge and Cairns 2012; Blow et al. 2006; Kawahara et al. 2007; Yang, Chrisman, and Weijer 2008). Thus, its potential function in the pathogenesis and progression of many neuropsychiatric diseases including schizophrenia has become a new trend in diagnostics and treatment. As post-mortem brain samples can provide straightforward information about miRNA dysregulation within the brain, for now, the only diagnostic tool is the biomarkers in the peripheral tissue samples from living subjects. Indeed, circulating miRNA levels in whole blood and plasma have shown potential as biomarkers of many disorders (Kawaguchi et al. 2016; Kichukova et al. 2015; Ripke et al. 2014) including schizophrenia (Kichukova et al. 2015; Wei et al. 2015; Ripke et al. 2014).

An analysis of copy number variants (CNV) shows that 22q11.2 deletion is associated with an increased risk for schizophrenia (Hiroi et al. 2013; Larsen et al. 2018). Furthermore, the 22q11.2 locus contains seven miRNA genes plus *DiGeorge syndrome critical region gene 8* (*DGCR8*). *DGCR8* encodes for a double-stranded-RNA-binding protein which is a crucial part of the miRNA biogenesis (Chen et al. 2012). Moreover, a genome-wide survey of miRNAs in rare CNV shows that the schizophrenia group is enriched with individuals having rare CNVs overlapping miRNA genes. To date, multiple lines of strong genetic evidence have suggested 108 genomic loci associated with schizophrenia containing 22 miRNA genes including *miR137* gene (Ripke et al. 2014). *miR137* is seen as a top genomic loci associated with schizophrenia in two genome-wide association studies with >10,000 samples (Hu et al. 2019; Merico et al. 2014). Another mRNA, *miR-9*, has been found to be dysregulated in neural progenitor cells of schizophrenia patients (Topol et al. 2016; Hu et al. 2019). Interestingly, target gene sets of *miR-137* and *miR-9-5p* are the main miRNA targetomes enhanced by schizophrenia risk genes (Ripke et al. 2014; Topol et al. 2016; Hu et al. 2019). Indeed, Wu et al., recently demonstrated that *miR-137* levels in peripheral blood cells may have the potential for diagnosing the early onset of schizophrenia (Wu et al. 2016). In another study which used binary regression analysis Ma et al. showed the association of *miR-22-3p*, *miR-92a-3p*, and *miR-137* with the schizophrenic phenotype (Ma et al. 2018). Analysis of the receiver operating characteristics (ROC) indicated that these three miRNAs could be used in combination as biomarkers for schizophrenia. Bioinformatic analyses of these genes and gene ontology enrichment showed that the combination of *miR-22-3p*, *miR-92a-3p*, and *miR-137* was tightly associated with synaptic structure and function, which play important roles in the etiology and pathophysiology of schizophrenia (Ma et al. 2018).

Recently Gardiner et al., described another locus, 14q32 which is an miRNA cluster, where more than 85% of the miRNAs expressed in this region showed a trend for downregulation in patients with schizophrenia (E. Gardiner et al. 2012). They examined miRNA expression in peripheral blood mononuclear cells from 112 patients with schizophrenia and 76 controls. They identified a significant reduction in 83 miRNAs in patients. Interestingly, a large subgroup consisting of 17 downregulated miRNAs is transcribed from a single imprinted locus at the maternally expressed *DLK1-DIO3* region on chromosome 14q32 (E. Gardiner et al. 2012). Thus, suggesting that altered expression of the miRNA from that pattern may be indicative of genetic or epigenetic dysregulation associated with the disease.

miRNAs negatively regulate target gene expression. Their biogenesis is tightly controlled by various factors including transcription factors that have been described before. Lui et al., in their study, explored the *TF-miRNA-30-target* gene axis as a novel biomarker that can be used for schizophrenia diagnosis and treatment monitoring (S. Liu et al. 2017). The qPCR analysis showed that an *early growth response protein 1* (*EGR1*) and *miR-30a-5p* were remarkably downregulated, while *neurogenic differentiation factor 1* (*NEUROD1*) was significantly upregulated in the blood from the patients in an acute psychotic state (S. Liu et al. 2017). Moreover, in the same study they investigated antipsychotic treatment that resulted in the elevation of *EGR1* and *miR-30a-5p* but the reduction of *NEUROD1*. Finally, receiver operating characteristic analysis demonstrated that the *EGR1-miR-30a-5p-NEUROD1* axis possessed greater diagnostic value than *miR-30a-5p* alone. Thus, *EGR1-miR-30a-5p-NEUROD1* axis could be a promising biomarker for diagnosis and treatment monitoring for patients in an acute psychotic state (S. Liu et al. 2017).

In the study of Wei et al, global plasma miRNAs were profiled in a test cohort of 164 patients with schizophrenia and 187 control subjects, using Solexa sequencing, TaqMan Low Density Array, and qPCR assays (Wei et al. 2015). They identified a new group of eight differentially expressed miRNAs (*miR-122, miR-130a, miR-130b, miR-193a-3p, miR-193b, miR-502-3p, miR-652* and *miR-886-5p*) in patients with schizophrenia (Wei et al. 2015). Furthermore, they noticed that an increased level of *miR-130b* and *miR193a-3p* in patients´ plasma disappeared after one year of treatment with aripiprazole and risperidone (Wei et al. 2015). Thus, they proposed *miR-130b* and *miR193a-3p* as potential biomarkers for the prognosis of schizophrenia treatment.

Many of the recent studies are focused on the clinical validation of the potential schizophrenia biomarkers. Sun et al., analyzed plasma levels of 10 miRNAs using qPCR in a cohort of 61 patients with schizophrenia and 62 healthy controls, as well as 25 patients specifically selected for a six-week antipsychotic treatment course (Sun et al. 2015). They found that a panel of miRNAs including *miR-30e, miR-181b, miR-34a, miR-346* and *miR-7* had significantly increased expression levels with significant combined diagnostic value. Furthermore, they investigated the response to pharmacological treatment, and they observed significant decreases in the expression levels of *miR-132, miR-181b, miR-432* and *miR-30e* (Sun et al. 2015). Finally, they checked the correlation between the improvement of the clinical symptoms with the changes in the expression levels of *miR-132, miR-181b, miR-212* and *miR-30e*. In summary, they concluded that *miR-30e, miR-181b, miR-34a, miR-346 and miR-7* combined as a panel are potentially useful non-invasive biomarkers for schizophrenia diagnosis and that *miR-132, miR-181b, miR-30e* and *miR-432* can be used as a potential indicator for symptomatology improvements, treatment responses and prognosis for patients affected with schizophrenia (Sun et al. 2015). A similar study has been performed by Sha Liu and collaborators. Using the extracted data from the literature on markers for schizophrenia published between 1990 and 2016 they performed a meta-analysis to examine miRNAs from peripheral blood mononuclear cells isolated from patients and healthy controls. The meta-analysis study was performed on a total number of 330 patients and 202 healthy controls. The results showed that levels of *miR-181b-5p, miR-21-5p, miR-195-5p, miR-137, miR-346* and *miR-34a-5p* in peripheral blood mononuclear cells present valuable diagnostic sensitivity in schizophrenia (Sha Liu et al. 2017).

Lai et al. examined the effect of hospitalization of the patients with schizophrenia on the expression level changes of seven miRNAs: *hsa-miR-34a, miR-449a, miR-564, miR-432, miR-548d, miR-572* and *miR-652*, that presented a signature as potential biomarkers for schizophrenia (Lai et al. 2011). The expression level of the above-listed miRNAs was not altered in the hospitalized patients with improvement, suggesting the miRNAs could be traits rather than state-dependent markers. Moreover, aberrant expression seen in the blood of *hsa-miR-34a* and *hsa-miR-548d* was not observed in the brain samples (Lai et al. 2011). Nevertheless, they found an age-dependent increase in *hsa-miR-34a* expression in Brodmann area 46 especially in the control group while the corresponding correlation in the blood was present only in the patients (Lai et al. 2011).

CONCLUSION

The search for blood biomarkers in mental illnesses such as schizophrenia is a topic that is currently rabid. However, studies in gene expression, with different techniques and greater or lesser precision have been in constant development for approximately 20 years. The biggest problems in detection of good blood gene expression markers in schizophrenia are, on the one hand, low sample numbers per study, which greatly reduces their value when analyzed in reference to the general population. On the other hand, the complexity of the phenotype of the patients with schizophrenia makes the identification difficult, since different patients can vary in numerous symptoms and signs of the disease. All in all, the future direction of studies of gene expression markers in the blood is to increase the number of patients and controls that are part of the evaluated sample. In addition, future studies must refine more precisely the endophenotype that they intend to study. Thus, this would avoid the inclusion of patients with different risk gene pools in the same study.

ACKNOWLEDGMENTS

We would like to thank Dr. Kelly Burke and Dr. Bruno Pinto for their help in reviewing the chapter.

REFERENCES

Aggarwal., B.B. (2003). "Signalling Pathways of the TNF Superfamily: A Double-Edged Sword." *Nature Reviews Immunology.*

Aliahmad., P., De La Torre., B., & Kaye., J. (2010). "Shared Dependence on the DNA-Binding Factor TOX for the Development of Lymphoid Tissue-Inducer Cell and NK Cell Lineages." *Nature Immunology* 11 (10): 945–52.

Amoli., M.M., Khatami., F., Arzaghi., S.M., Enayati., S., & Nejatisafa., A.A. (2019). "Over-Expression of TGF-B1 Gene in Medication Free Schizophrenia." *Psychoneuroendocrinology* 99 (January): 265–70.

Andrews., Z.B. (2011). "Central Mechanisms Involved in the Orexigenic Actions of Ghrelin." *Peptides.*

Beveren., N.JM., van, Buitendijk., G.H.S., Swagemakers., S., Krab., L.C., Röder., C., de Haan., L., van der Spek., P., & Elgersma., Y. (2012). "Marked Reduction of AKT1 Expression and Deregulation of AKT1-Associated Pathways in Peripheral Blood Mononuclear Cells of Schizophrenia Patients." *PLoS ONE* 7 (2).

Beveridge., N..J, & Cairns., M.J. (2012). "MicroRNA Dysregulation in Schizophrenia." *Neurobiology of Disease.*

Blow., M.J., Grocock., R.J., van Dongen., S., Enright., A.J., Dicks., E., Futreal., P.A., Wooster., R., & Stratton., M.R. (2006). "RNA Editing of Human MicroRNAs." *Genome Biology* 7 (4).

Boneberg., E..M, Von Seydlitz., E., Pröpster., K., Watzl., H., Rockstroh., B., & Illges., H. (2006). "D3 Dopamine Receptor MRNA Is Elevated in T Cells of Schizophrenic Patients Whereas D4 Dopamine Receptor MRNA Is Reduced in CD4+-T Cells." *Journal of Neuroimmunology* 173 (1–2): 180–87.

Bowden., N.A., Weidenhofer., J., Scott., R.J., Schall., U., Todd., J., Michie., P.T., & Tooney., A. (2006). "Preliminary Investigation of Gene Expression Profiles in Peripheral Blood Lymphocytes in Schizophrenia." *Schizophrenia Research* 82 (2–3): 175–83.

Chase., K.A., Feiner., B., Rosen., C., Gavin., D.P., & Sharma., P. (2016). "Characterization of Peripheral Cannabinoid Receptor Expression and Clinical Correlates in Schizophrenia." *Psychiatry Research* 245 (November): 346–53.

Chen., Z., Wu., J., Yang., C., Fan., P., Balazs., L., Jiao., Y., Lu., M., et al. (2012). "DiGeorge Syndrome Critical Region 8 (DGCR8) Protein-Mediated MicroRNA Biogenesis Is Essential for Vascular Smooth Muscle Cell Development in Mice." *Journal of Biological Chemistry* 287 (23): 19018–28.

Cho., K.H.T., Xu., B., Blenkiron., C., & Fraser., M. (2019). "Emerging Roles of MiRNAs in Brain Development and Perinatal Brain Injury." *Frontiers in Physiology* 10 (MAR).

Chuang., J.C., & Zigman., J.M. (2010). "Ghrelin's Roles in Stress, Mood, and Anxiety Regulation." *International Journal of Peptides*.

DeRosse., P., Kaplan., A., Burdick., K.E., Lencz., T., & Malhotra., A.K. (2010). "Cannabis Use Disorders in Schizophrenia: Effects on Cognition and Symptoms." *Schizophrenia Research* 120 (1–3): 95–100.

Dmitriev., S.E., Terenin., I.M., Andreev., D.E., Ivanov., P.A., Dunaevsky., J.E., Merrick., W.C., & Shatsky., I.N. (2010). "GTP-Independent TRNA Delivery to the Ribosomal P-Site by a Novel Eukaryotic Translation Factor." *Journal of Biological Chemistry* 285 (35): 26779–87.

Drexhage., R.C., Knijff., E.M., Padmos., R.C., Van Der Heul-Nieuwenhuijzen., L., Beumer., W., Versnel., M.A., & Drexhage., H.A. (2010). "The Mononuclear Phagocyte System and Its Cytokine Inflammatory Networks in Schizophrenia and Bipolar Disorder." *Expert Review of Neurotherapeutics*.

Fallah., H., Azari., I., Neishabouri., S.M., Oskooei., K., Taheri., M., & Ghafouri-Fard., S. (2019). "Sex-Specific up-Regulation of LncRNAs

in Peripheral Blood of Patients with Schizophrenia." *Scientific Reports* 9 (1).
Fineberg., S.K., Kosik., K.S., & Davidson., B.L. (2009). "MicroRNAs Potentiate Neural Development." *Neuron*.
Gallego., J.A., Blanco., E.A., Husain-Krautter., S., Madeline Fagen., E., Moreno-Merino., P., del Ojo-Jiménez., J.A., Ahmed., A., Rothstein., T.L., Lencz., T., & Malhotra., A.K. (2018). "Cytokines in Cerebrospinal Fluid of Patients with Schizophrenia Spectrum Disorders: New Data and an Updated Meta-Analysis." *Schizophrenia Research* 202 (December): 64–71.
Gardiner., E., Beveridge., N.J., Wu., J.Q., Carr., V., Scott., R.J., Tooney., P.A., & Cairns., M.J. (2012). "Imprinted DLK1-DIO3 Region of 14q32 Defines a Schizophrenia-Associated MiRNA Signature in Peripheral Blood Mononuclear Cells." *Molecular Psychiatry* 17 (8): 827–40.
Gardiner., E.J., Cairns., M.J., Liu., B., Beveridge., N.J., Carr., V., Kelly., B., Scott., R.J., & Tooney., P.A. (2013). "Gene Expression Analysis Reveals Schizophrenia-Associated Dysregulation of Immune Pathways in Peripheral Blood Mononuclear Cells." *Journal of Psychiatric Research* 47 (4): 425–37.
Gibb., J., Hayley., S., Gandhi., R., Poulter., M.O., & Anisman., H. (2008). "Synergistic and Additive Actions of a Psychosocial Stressor and Endotoxin Challenge: Circulating and Brain Cytokines, Plasma Corticosterone and Behavioral Changes in Mice." *Brain, Behavior, and Immunity* 22 (4): 573–89.
Gilabert-Juan., J., López-Campos., G., Sebastiá-Ortega., N., Guara-Ciurana., S., Ruso-Julve., F., Prieto., C., Crespo-Facorro., B., Sanjuán., J., & Moltó., M.D. (2019). "Time Dependent Expression of the Blood Biomarkers EIF2D and TOX in Patients with Schizophrenia." *Brain, Behavior, and Immunity* 80 (August): 909–15.
Glatt., S.J., Stone., W.S., Nossova., N., Liew., C-C, Seidman., LJ, & Tsuang., MT. (2011). "Similarities and Differences in Peripheral Blood Gene-Expression Signatures of Individuals with Schizophrenia and Their First-Degree Biological Relatives." *American Journal of*

Medical Genetics Part B: Neuropsychiatric Genetics 156 (8): 869–87.

Grayson., D.R., Chen., Y., Costa., E., Dong., E., Guidotti., A., Kundakovic., M., & Sharma., R.P. (2006). "The Human Reelin Gene: Transcription Factors (+), Repressors (-) and the Methylation Switch (+/-) in Schizophrenia." *Pharmacology and Therapeutics*.

Haghighatfard., A., Andalib., S., Amini Faskhodi., M., Sadeghi., S., Ghaderi., A.H., Moradkhani., S., Rostampour., J., et al. (2018). "Gene Expression Study of Mitochondrial Complex I in Schizophrenia and Paranoid Personality Disorder." *World Journal of Biological Psychiatry* 19 (sup3): S133–46.

Heringa., S.M., Begemann., M.J.H., Goverde., A.J., & Sommer., I.E.C. (2015). "Sex Hormones and Oxytocin Augmentation Strategies in Schizophrenia: A Quantitative Review." *Schizophrenia Research*.

Hess., J.L., Tylee., D.S., Barve., R., de Jong., S., Ophoff., R.A., Kumarasinghe., N., Tooney., P., et al. (2016). "Transcriptome-Wide Mega-Analyses Reveal Joint Dysregulation of Immunologic Genes and Transcription Regulators in Brain and Blood in Schizophrenia." *Schizophrenia Research* 176 (2–3): 114–24.

Hiroi., N., Takahashi., T., Hishimoto., A., Izumi., T., Boku., S., & Hiramoto., T. (2013). "Copy Number Variation at 22q11.2: From Rare Variants to Common Mechanisms of Developmental Neuropsychiatric Disorders." *Molecular Psychiatry*.

Hoseth., E.Z., Ueland., T., Dieset., I., Birnbaum., R., Shin., J.H., Kleinman., J.E., Hyde., T.M., et al. (2017). "A Study of TNF Pathway Activation in Schizophrenia and Bipolar Disorder in Plasma and Brain Tissue." *Schizophrenia Bulletin* 43 (4): 881–90.

Hu., Z., Gao., S., Lindberg., D., Panja., D., Wakabayashi., Y., Li., K., Kleinman., J.E., Zhu., J., & Li., Z. (2019). "Temporal Dynamics of MiRNAs in Human DLPFC and Its Association with MiRNA Dysregulation in Schizophrenia." *Translational Psychiatry* 9 (1): 1–17.

Ilani., T. (2001). "A Peripheral Marker for Schizophrenia: Increased Levels of D3 Dopamine Receptor MRNA in Blood Lymphocytes."

Proceedings of the National Academy of Sciences 98 (2): 625–28.

Jerlhag., E., Egecioglu., E., Landgren., S., Salomé., N., Heilig., M., Moechars., D., Datta., R., Perrissoud., D., Dickson., S.L., & Engel., J.A. (2009). "Requirement of Central Ghrelin Signaling for Alcohol Reward." *Proceedings of the National Academy of Sciences of the United States of America* 106 (27): 11318–23.

Kawaguchi., T., Komatsu., S., Ichikawa., D., Tsujiura., M., Takeshita., H., Hirajima., S., Miyamae., M., et al. (2016). "Circulating MicroRNAS: A next-Generation Clinical Biomarker for Digestive System Cancers." *International Journal of Molecular Sciences*.

Kawahara., Y., Zinshteyn., B., Chendrimada., T.P., Shiekhattar., R., & Nishikura., K. (2007). "RNA Editing of the MicroRNA-151 Precursor Blocks Cleavage by the Dicer - TRBP Complex." *EMBO Reports* 8 (8): 763–69.

Kichukova., T.M., Popov., N.T., Ivanov., H.Y., & Vachev., T.I. (2015). "Circulating MicroRNAs as a Novel Class of Potential Diagnostic Biomarkers in Neuropsychiatric Disorders." *Folia Medica*.

Kida., Y., Shiraishi., T., & Ogura., T. (2004). "Identification of Chick and Mouse Daam1 and Daam2 Genes and Their Expression Patterns in the Central Nervous System." *Developmental Brain Research* 153 (1): 143–50.

Kluge., M., Schüssler., P., Bleninger., P., Kleyer., S., Uhr., M., Weikel., J.C., Yassouridis., A., Zuber., V., & Steiger., A. (2008). "Ghrelin Alone or Co-Administered with GHRH or CRH Increases Non-REM Sleep and Decreases REM Sleep in Young Males." *Psychoneuroendocrinology* 33 (4): 497–506.

Kojima., M., Hosoda., H., Date., Y., Nakazato., M., Matsuo., H., & Kangawa., K. (1999). "Ghrelin Is a Growth-Hormone-Releasing Acylated Peptide from Stomach." *Nature* 402 (6762): 656–60.

Koren., A., Polak., P., Nemesh., J., Michaelson., J.J., Sebat., J., Sunyaev., S.R., & McCarroll., S.A. (2012). "Differential Relationship of DNA Replication Timing to Different Forms of Human Mutation and Variation." *American Journal of Human Genetics* 91 (6): 1033–40.

Kozłowska., E., Agier., J., Wysokiński., A., Łucka., A., Sobierajska., K., &

Brzezińska-Błaszczyk., E. (2019). "The Expression of Toll-like Receptors in Peripheral Blood Mononuclear Cells Is Altered in Schizophrenia." *Psychiatry Research* 272 (February): 540–50.

Kumarasinghe., N., Beveridge., N.J., Gardiner., E., Scott., R.J., Yasawardene., S., Perera., A., Mendis., J., Suriyakumara., K., Schall., U., & Tooney., P.A. (2013). "Gene Expression Profiling in Treatment-Naive Schizophrenia Patients Identifies Abnormalities in Biological Pathways Involving AKT1 That Are Corrected by Antipsychotic Medication." *International Journal of Neuropsychopharmacology* 16 (7): 1483–1503.

Kuzman., M.R., Medved., V., Terzic., J., & Krainc., D. (2009). "Genome-Wide Expression Analysis of Peripheral Blood Identifies Candidate Biomarkers for Schizophrenia." *Journal of Psychiatric Research* 43 (13): 1073–77.

Kwak., Y.T., Koo., M.S., Choi., C.H., & Sunwoo., I.N. (2001). "Change of Dopamine Receptor MRNA Expression in Lymphocyte of Schizophrenic Patients." *BMC Medical Genetics* 2 (March): 3.

Lai., C.Y., Yu., S.L., Hsieh., M.H., Chen., C.H., Chen., H.Y., Wen., C.C, Huang., Y..H., et al. (2011). "MicroRNA Expression Aberration as Potential Peripheral Blood Biomarkers for Schizophrenia." Edited by Monica Uddin. *PLoS ONE* 6 (6): e21635.

Larsen., K.M., Pellegrino., G., Birknow., M.R., Kjær., T..N, Baaré., W.F.C., Didriksen., M., Olsen., L., Werge., T., Mørup., M., & Siebner., H.R. (2018). "22q11.2 Deletion Syndrome Is Associated With Impaired Auditory Steady-State Gamma Response." *Schizophrenia Bulletin* 44 (2): 388–97.

Lee., R.C., Feinbaum., R.L., & Ambros., V. (1993). "The C. Elegans Heterochronic Gene Lin-4 Encodes Small RNAs with Antisense Complementarity to Lin-14." *Cell* 75 (5): 843–54.

Leirer., D.J., Iyegbe., C.O., Di Forti., M., Patel., H., Carra., E., Fraietta., S., Colizzi., M., et al. (2019). "Differential Gene Expression Analysis in Blood of First Episode Psychosis Patients." *Schizophrenia Research* 209 (July): 88–97.

Liu., L., Jia., F., Yuan., G., Chen., Z., Yao., J., Li., H., & Fang., C. (2010).

"Tyrosine Hydroxylase, Interleukin-1β and Tumor Necrosis Factor-α Are Overexpressed in Peripheral Blood Mononuclear Cells from Schizophrenia Patients as Determined by Semi-Quantitative Analysis." *Psychiatry Research* 176 (1): 1–7.

Liu., S., Zhang., F., Shugart., Y.Y., Yang., L., Li., X., Liu., Z., Sun., N., et al. (2017). "The Early Growth Response Protein 1-MiR-30a-5p-Neurogenic Differentiation Factor 1 Axis as a Novel Biomarker for Schizophrenia Diagnosis and Treatment Monitoring." *Translational Psychiatry* 7 (1).

Liu., Sha., Zhang., F., Wang., X., Shugart., Y.Y., Zhao., Y., Li., X., Liu., Z., et al. (2017). "Diagnostic Value of Blood-Derived MicroRNAs for Schizophrenia: Results of a Meta-Analysis and Validation." *Scientific Reports* 7 (1): 1–10.

Long., Y., Wang., X., Youmans., D.T., & Cech., T.R. (2017). "How Do LncRNAs Regulate Transcription?" *Science Advances*.

Ma., J., Shang., S., Wang., J., Zhang., T., Nie., F., Song., X., Heping Zhao, Zhu., C., Zhang., R., & Hao., D. (2018). "Identification of MiR-22-3p, MiR-92a-3p, and MiR-137 in Peripheral Blood as Biomarker for Schizophrenia." *Psychiatry Research* 265 (July): 70–76.

Mas., S., Gassó., P., Ritter., M.A., Malagelada., C., Bernardo., M., & Lafuente., A. (2015). "Pharmacogenetic Predictor of Extrapyramidal Symptoms Induced by Antipsychotics: Multilocus Interaction in the MTOR Pathway." *European Neuropsychopharmacology* 25 (1): 51–59.

Mehler-Wex., C., Duvigneau., J.C., Hartl., R.T., Ben-Shachar., D., Warnke., A., & Gerlach., M. (2006). "Increased MRNA Levels of the Mitochondrial Complex I 75-KDa Subunit: A Potential Peripheral Marker of Early Onset Schizophrenia?" *European Child and Adolescent Psychiatry* 15 (8): 504–7.

Meltzer., H.Y. (1999). "The Role of Serotonin in Antipsychotic Drug Action." *Neuropsychopharmacology* 21 (2 Suppl): 106S-115S.

Merico., D., Costain., G., Butcher., N.J., Warnica., W., Ogura., L., Alfred., S.E., Brzustowicz., L.M., & Bassett., A.S.. (2014). "MicroRNA Dysregulation, Gene Networks and Risk for Schizophrenia in

22q11.2 Deletion Syndrome." *Frontiers in Neurology* 5 (NOV).

Moreno-Küstner., B., Martín., C., & Pastor., L. (2018). "Prevalence of Psychotic Disorders and Its Association with Methodological Issues. A Systematic Review and Meta-Analyses." *PLoS ONE*.

Moretti., P.N., Ota., V.K., Gouvea., E.S., Pedrini., M., Santoro., M.L., Talarico., F., Spindola., L.M., et al. (2018). "Accessing Gene Expression in Treatment-Resistant Schizophrenia." *Molecular Neurobiology* 55 (8): 7000–7008.

Nakata., S., Yoshino., Y., Okita., M., Kawabe., K., Yamazaki., K., Ozaki., Y., Mori., Y., Ochi., S., Iga., J., & Ueno., S. (2019). "Differential Expression of the Ghrelin-Related MRNAs GHS-R1a, GHS-R1b, and MBOAT4 in Japanese Patients with Schizophrenia." *Psychiatry Research* 272 (February): 334–39.

Okazaki., S., Boku., S., Otsuka., I., Mouri., K., Aoyama., S., Shiroiwa., K., Sora., I., et al. (2016). "The Cell Cycle-Related Genes as Biomarkers for Schizophrenia." *Progress in Neuro-Psychopharmacology and Biological Psychiatry* 70 (October): 85–91.

Ota., V.K., Moretti., P.N., Santoro., M.L., Talarico., F., Spindola., L.M., Xavier., G., Carvalho., C.M., et al. (2019). "Gene Expression over the Course of Schizophrenia: From Clinical High-Risk for Psychosis to Chronic Stages." *Npj Schizophrenia* 5 (1): 5.

Ota., V.K., Noto., C., Santoro., M.L., Spindola., L.M., Gouvea., E.S., Carvalho., C.M., Santos., C.M., et al. (2015). "Increased Expression of NDEL1 and MBP Genes in the Peripheral Blood of Antipsychotic-Naïve Patients with First-Episode Psychosis." *European Neuropsychopharmacology* 25 (12): 2416–25.

Pei., L., & Wallace., D.C. (2018). "Mitochondrial Etiology of Neuropsychiatric Disorders." *Biological Psychiatry*.

Proitsi., P., Li., T., Hamilton., G., Di Forti., M., Collier., D., Killick., R., Chen., R., et al. (2008). "Positional Pathway Screen of Wnt Signaling Genes in Schizophrenia: Association with DKK4." *Biological Psychiatry* 63 (1): 13–16.

Rabin., R.A., Zakzanis., K.K., & George., T.P. (2011). "The Effects of Cannabis Use on Neurocognition in Schizophrenia: A Meta-

Analysis." *Schizophrenia Research* 128 (1–3): 111–16.
Ripke., S., Neale., B.M., Corvin., A., Walters., J.T.R., Farh., K.H., Holmans., P.A., Lee., P., et al. (2014). "Biological Insights from 108 Schizophrenia-Associated Genetic Loci." *Nature* 511 (7510): 421–27.
Smith., R.S. (1992). "A Comprehensive Macrophage-T-Lymphocyte Theory of Schizophrenia." *Medical Hypotheses* 39 (3): 248–57.
Smith., R.S., & Maes., M. (1995). "The Macrophage-T-Lymphocyte Theory of Schizophrenia: Additional Evidence." *Medical Hypotheses* 45 (2): 135–41.
Staal., S.P. (1987). "Molecular Cloning of the Akt Oncogene and Its Human Homologues AKT1 and AKT2: Amplification of AKT1 in a Primary Human Gastric Adenocarcinoma." *Proceedings of the National Academy of Sciences of the United States of America* 84 (14): 5034–37.
Suárez-Pinilla., P., Roiz-Santiañez., R., Ortiz-García de la Foz., V., Guest., P.C., Ayesa-Arriola., R., Córdova-Palomera., A., Tordesillas-Gutierrez., D., & Crespo-Facorro., B. (2015). "Brain Structural and Clinical Changes after First Episode Psychosis: Focus on Cannabinoid Receptor 1 Polymorphisms." *Psychiatry Research - Neuroimaging* 233 (2): 112–19.
Sun., Y., Zhang., J., Niu., W., Guo., W., Song., H.T., Li., H.Y., Fan., H.M., et al. (2015). "A Preliminary Analysis of MicroRNA as Potential Clinical Biomarker for Schizophrenia." *American Journal of Medical Genetics, Part B: Neuropsychiatric Genetics* 168 (3): 170–78.
Takahashi., M., Hayashi., H., Watanabe., Y., Sawamura., K., Fukui., N., Watanabe., J., Kitajima., T., et al. (2010). "Diagnostic Classification of Schizophrenia by Neural Network Analysis of Blood-Based Gene Expression Signatures." *Schizophrenia Research* 119 (1–3): 210–18.
Taurines., R., Thome., J., Duvigneau., J.C., Forbes-Robertson., S., Yang., L., Klampfl., K., Romanos., J., Müller., S., Gerlach., M., & Mehler-Wex., C. (2010). "Expression Analyses of the Mitochondrial Complex i 75-KDa Subunit in Early Onset Schizophrenia and Autism Spectrum Disorder: Increased Levels as a Potential Biomarker for Early Onset Schizophrenia." *European Child and Adolescent*

Psychiatry 19 (5): 441–48.

Tecchio., C., Micheletti., A., & Cassatella., M.A. (2014). "Neutrophil-Derived Cytokines: Facts beyond Expression." *Frontiers in Immunology*.

Topol., A., Zhu., S., Hartley., B.J., English., J., Hauberg., M.E., Tran., N., Rittenhouse., C.A., et al. (2016). "Dysregulation of MiRNA-9 in a Subset of Schizophrenia Patient-Derived Neural Progenitor Cells." *Cell Reports* 15 (5): 1024–36.

Ukkola-Vuoti., L., Torniainen-Holm., M., Ortega-Alonso., A., Sinha., V., Tuulio-Henriksson., A., Paunio., T., Lönnqvist., J., Suvisaari., J., & Hennah., W. (2019). "Gene Expression Changes Related to Immune Processes Associate with Cognitive Endophenotypes of Schizophrenia." *Progress in Neuro-Psychopharmacology and Biological Psychiatry* 88 (January): 159–67.

Upthegrove., R., Manzanares-Teson., N., & Barnes., N.M. (2014). "Cytokine Function in Medication-Naive First Episode Psychosis: A Systematic Review and Meta-Analysis." *Schizophrenia Research* 155 (1–3): 101–8.

Vogel., M., Pfeifer., S., Schaub., R.T., Grabe., H.J., Barnow., S., Freyberger., H.J., & Cascorbi., I. (2004). "Decreased Levels of Dopamine D3 Receptor MRNA in Schizophrenic and Bipolar Patients." *Neuropsychobiology* 50 (4): 305–10.

Wei., H., Yuan., Y., Liu., S., Wang., C., Yang., F., Lu., Z., Wang., C., et al. (2015). "Detection of Circulating MiRNA Levels in Schizophrenia." *American Journal of Psychiatry* 172 (11): 1141–47.

Wu., S., Zhang., R., Nie., F., Wang., X., Jiang., C., Liu., M., Valenzuela., R.K., Liu., W., Shi., Y., & Ma., J. (2016). "MicroRNA-137 Inhibits EFNB2 Expression Affected by a Genetic Variant and Is Expressed Aberrantly in Peripheral Blood of Schizophrenia Patients." *EBioMedicine* 12 (October): 133–42.

Yang., X., Chrisman., H., & Weijer., C.J. (2008). "PDGF Signalling Controls the Migration of Mesoderm Cells during Chick Gastrulation by Regulating N-Cadherin Expression." *Development* 135 (21): 3521–30.

Yee., J.Y., Nurjono., M., Ng., W.Y., Teo., S.R., Lee., T.S., & Lee., J. (2017). "Peripheral Blood Gene Expression of Acute Phase Proteins in People with First Episode Psychosis." *Brain, Behavior, and Immunity* 65 (October): 337–41.

Yu., H., Bi., W., Liu., C., Zhao., Y., Zhang., J.F., Zhang., D., & Yue., W. (2014). "Protein-Interaction-Network-Based Analysis for Genome-Wide Association Analysis of Schizophrenia in Han Chinese Population." *Journal of Psychiatric Research* 50 (1): 73–78.

Zvara., Á., Szekeres., G., Janka., Z., Kelemen., J.Z., Cimmer., C., Sántha., M., & Puskás., L.G. (2005). "Over-Expression of Dopamine D2 Receptor and Inwardly Rectifying Potassium Channel Genes in Drug-Naive Schizophrenic Peripheral Blood Lymphocytes as Potential Diagnostic Markers." *Disease Markers* 21 (2): 61–69.

In: Schizophrenia
Editor: Bojan Sterenborg
ISBN: 978-1-53618-144-9
© 2020 Nova Science Publishers, Inc.

Chapter 3

THE ROLE OF INTERNALIZED STIGMA IN THE FEAR OF NEGATIVE EVALUATION IN PATIENTS WITH SCHIZOPHRENIA

Ana Fresán[1,]*, Rebeca Robles-García[2], María Yoldi-Negrete[1], J. Nicolás Martínez-López[1], Carlos-Alfonso Tovilla-Zárate[3], Tania Real[2], Ricardo Saracco-Alvarez[1] and Eduardo Madrigal[4]

[1]Subdirección de Investigaciones Clínicas.
Instituto Nacional de Psiquiatría Ramón de la Fuente Muñíz,
Ciudad de México, México
[2]Centro de Investigación en Salud Mental Global.
Instituto Nacional de Psiquiatría Ramón de la Fuente Muñíz,
Ciudad de México, México
[3]Universidad Juárez Autónoma de Tabasco,
División Académica Multidisciplinaria de Comalcalco,
Comalcalco, Tabasco, México
[4]Dirección General. Instituto Nacional de Psiquiatría Ramón de la Fuente Muñíz, Ciudad de México, México

---

* Corresponding author: Ana Fresán, PsyD, PhD, Instituto Nacional de Psiquiatría Ramón de la Fuente Muñíz, Calz. México-Xochimilco 101, Mexico City, 14370, Mexico, Telephone: (5255) 41605069, E-mail: fresan@imp.edu.mx; a_fresan@yahoo.com.mx.

ABSTRACT

Introduction: Fear is conceived as a normal reaction to threat and is related to a function of survival. However, some people may experience an intense and persistent fear or embarrassment in social situations where they are under the observation or examination of others. This may reflect a core feature of social anxiety, a disorder which interferes with everyday activities. Social anxiety and subthreshold symptoms, defined as an excessive fear of negative evaluation (FNE) from others leading to avoidance of social interactions, is a common comorbid condition among people with schizophrenia, with a deleterious effect on global functioning and quality of life.

Fear of negative evaluation might emerge from several factors, such as biases in cognitive processing, inadequate self-perception in relation to others, and even variables related to the individual's clinical background such as age of onset, delay in specialized treatment and symptom severity. Nevertheless, as its expression is related to the appreciation of others, factors outside the individuals background are necessary to be considered.

Schizophrenia is one of the most stigmatized mental disorders worldwide. The negative public attitudes and beliefs toward the disorder have negative impact on early diagnosis and adequate specialized treatment of the disorder. Also, another consequence may be the internalization of these stigmatizing conceptions, leading to low self-esteem, hopelessness about treatment and recovery.

Some patients may be more susceptible to the criticism and negative attitudes of others toward the disorder they suffer and, eventually, may express symptoms of social anxiety such as fear of negative evaluation as a response to public and internalized stigma.

Therefore, the present study aimed to determine the role of internalized stigma in the presence and severity of fear of negative evaluation in patients with schizophrenia. Specifically, we hypothesized that patients with prominent FNE will report more internalized stigma and that a higher perceived discrimination (internalized stigma dimension) will be the most important predictor of prominent FNE in patients with schizophrenia. We further hypothesized that groups differences will be observed in symptom severity at the time of the study, with more pronounced negative and affective symptoms in the group of patients with prominent fear of negative evaluation.

Method: Two-hundred and sixty-nine patients with DSM-IV-TR diagnosis of schizophrenia according to the Structured Clinical Interview for DSM-IV Axis I Disorders (SCID-I) were recruited. Symptom severity at the time of the study were rated using the 5-dimensional model of the Positive and Negative Syndrome Scale (PANSS). The King's Internalized

Stigma Scale (ISS) was used for the assessment of three main areas of internalized stigma: perceived discrimination, disclosure about mental illness and positive aspects of mental illness. Finally, for the evaluation of fear of negative evaluation, the Brief Fear of Negative Evaluation Scale – Revised (BFNE-II) was used.

The upper quartile (75%) of the BFNE-II total score was used to divide the sample in those patients with prominent FNE and those with absent/mild FNE. Comparative analyses between groups were performed and a multivariate logistic regression analysis was used to determine risk factors associated to prominent FNE in patients with schizophrenia.

Results: Men accounted for 68.4% (n = 184) of the sample with a mean age of 37 years (S.D. = 10.7). Most of the patients were unemployed (72.1, n = 194) and single (98.9%, n = 266). Age of illness onset was reported at 24.2 (S.D. = 7.) years with 56.1% (n = 151) with a history of previous psychiatric hospitalizations. Using the proposed cut-off point 26.4% (n = 71) of the patients were classified in the group of prominent FNE. Demographic features were similar between FNE groups as well as current psychotic symptomatology assessed with the 5-dimensional model of the PANSS (p > 0.05). A greater number of patients with prominent FNE reported previous psychiatric hospitalizations (61.1% vs. 42.3%, p = 0.006). The three dimensions that comprise internalized stigma and its total score was significantly higher in patients with prominent FNE (p < 0.01) and the dimensions of perceived discrimination and positive aspects of mental illness were predictors of prominent FNE inpatients with schizophrenia (OR = 1.0, 95% C.I. = 1.05 - 1.13 and OR = 1.1, 95% C.I. = 1.08 - 1.30 respectively).

Discussion: Internalized stigma has been associated with higher levels of anxiety in patients with schizophrenia. Although the present study did not determine a definite comorbid social anxiety disorder, our results showed that some patients may have a greater predisposition to fear of negative evaluation in the context of internalization of public stigma. Future studies should address the presence and severity of fear of negative evaluation and internalized stigma in patients with schizophrenia and confidently be differentiated from characteristic symptoms of schizophrenia (as positive and negative symptoms). This, in order to provide effective treatment, pharmacologic and therapeutic for both: anxiety symptoms generated by the fear of negative evaluation and the symptoms of schizophrenia; and thus, reduce as far as possible the social deterioration that the patient could present when having both conditions.

Keywords: schizophrenia, fear of negative evaluation, internalized stigma, anxiety

INTRODUCTION

Fear is conceived as a normal reaction to threat and is related to a function of survival and is evoked when the organism is under a real or imaginary threat (Gullone, 2000; Mobbs, 2018). To understand fear, it is important to examine the natural world and those stimuli that generate it. Social evaluations are a natural part of the social interactions of a human being. However, for some individuals, these evaluations represent a source of distress originating an intense and persistent fear or embarrassment when under the observation or examination of others.

Fear of negative evaluation (FNE) is defined as a threat related to an extreme apprehension of others' negative evaluations or judgements, avoidance of situations where evaluation is likely to happen and the expectation that others would evaluate oneself negatively (Reichenberger, et. al., 2018). FNE is a core feature of social anxiety (American Psychiatric Association, 2013), a disabling mental disorder associated with high distress and difficulties in everyday activities across educational, occupational, interpersonal and social domains (Michail & Birchwoon, 2014; Michail, et. al., 2017). Social anxiety and subthreshold symptoms that lead to the avoidance of social interactions with a deleterious effect on global functioning and quality of life, is a common comorbid condition among people with schizophrenia, with an estimated prevalence rate between 19% and 31% in individuals diagnosed with a psychotic disorder attending outpatient psychiatric services (McEnery, et. al., 2019).

Some cognitive theories of social anxiety emphasize the role of negative self-appraisals, the tendency to see oneself as responsible for other people's discomfort and the distress that arises from concerns of being negatively judged by others (Rector, et. al., 2006). Individuals with schizophrenia frequently display shyness, poor socialization and a history of problems with social interactions. In many cases, these social difficulties can be observed since childhood (Braga, et. al., 2005) and be related to prodromal features of the disease. In others, they can be the effect of the insidious manifestation and maintenance of positive and negative symptoms as well as emotional difficulties that may arise during the clinical course of the disorder (Lysaker, et. al., 2010; Kinoshita, et. al., 2011). However, the apprehension about receiving negative evaluation from others might have an important role in this sensitivity or aversiveness towards interpersonal social interactions in individuals with schizophrenia.

Social anxiety symptoms, in the context of fear of negative evaluation, might emerge from several factors, such as biases in cognitive processing, inadequate self-perception in relation to others, and even variables related to the individual's clinical background such as age of onset, delay in specialized treatment and symptom severity (Bosanac, et al., 2016; Aikawa, et al., 2018). Nevertheless, as its expression is related to the appreciation of others, factors outside the individuals' background must necessarily be considered.

Schizophrenia is one of the most stigmatized mental disorders worldwide, with misconceptions about the disease related to dangerousness, violence and unpredictability (Fresán & Robles-García, 2011). These negative public attitudes and beliefs toward the disorder have an important and negative impact in the persons affected by this illness. In addition, there can be internalization of these stigmatizing conceptions, leading to low self-esteem, hopelessness about treatment and recovery and even application of stigmatizing attitudes and behaviors to oneself (self-contempt, isolation, self-aggression).

Although not all patients internalize public stigma, there may be others that are more susceptible to the criticism and negative attitude of others toward the disorder they suffer and eventually may express significant fear of negative evaluation as a response to public and internalized stigma (Pallanti, et al., 2004).

Therefore, the present study aimed to determine the role of internalized stigma in the presence and severity of fear of negative evaluation in patients with schizophrenia. Specifically, we hypothesized that patients with prominent FNE will report more internalized stigma and that a higher perceived discrimination (internalized stigma dimension) will be the most important predictor of prominent FNE in patients with schizophrenia. We further hypothesized that groups differences will be observed in some clinical features of the disorder (age of illness onset, duration of untreated psychosis and history of psychiatric hospitalizations) and symptom severity at the time of the study with more pronounced negative and affective symptoms in the group of patients with prominent fear of negative evaluation.

METHODS

The present study was approved by the research ethic board of the *Instituto Nacional de Psiquiatría Ramón de la Fuente Muñíz* (INPRFM), a highly specialized psychiatric facility in Mexico City. Patient recruitment was done in accordance to a non-probabilistic sample approach. All patients willing to participate and who met inclusion and exclusion criteria were recruited. Before enrollment, all patients gave their written informed consent to participate after the aims of the study were fully explained.

Participants

Two-hundred and sixty-nine patients with DSM-IV-TR diagnosis of schizophrenia according to the Structured Clinical Interview for DSM-IV Axis I Disorders (SCID-I) were included (First, et al., 1997). All patients were under antipsychotic treatment and were treated at the outpatient services at the INPRFM. Patients were excluded from the study if they had any concomitant medical or neurological disease according to a face-to-face interview and medical records, if they were agitated during the assessment or were clinically unstable, in accordance to treating psychiatrist, that impeded the interview.

Assessment Procedures

Psychotic symptom severity was assessed with the *Positive and Negative Syndrome Scale* (PANSS) (Kay, et al., 1990). The PANSS includes 30 symptoms, measured at present and over the past month on a scale from 1 = absent to 7 = extreme. The dimensional model of the PANSS positive, negative, cognitive, excitement and depression/anxiety subscales validated in Mexican population was used (Fresán, et al., 2005).

The King's Internalized Stigma Scale (ISS) (King, et al., 2007) validated in Mexican population (Flores-Reynoso, et al., 2011) was used for the assessment of three main areas of internalized stigma: perceived discrimination, disclosure about mental illness and positive aspects of mental illness. The scale comprise 28 self-report items rated on a Likert scale from 0 = strongly agree to 4 = strongly disagree.

Finally, for the evaluation of fear of negative evaluation, the Brief Fear of Negative Evaluation Scale – Revised (BFNE-II) was used (Carleton, et al., 2006; Carleton, et al., 2007; Leary, 1983). The scale comprise 12 self-report items assessed in a Likert frequency scale from 0 = Never/almost never to 4 = Always/almost always. This scale showed adequate internal consistency and construct validity for its use in Mexican population (Robles-García, et al., 2012). The upper quartile (75%) of the BFNE-II total score was used to divide the sample in those patients with prominent FNE and those with absent/mild FNE.

Statistical Analysis

All statistical procedures were performed using the SPSS statistical software version 21. Demographic and clinical features were described with frequencies and percentages for categorical variables and with means and standard deviations (S.D.) for continuous variables. Chi square tests ($x2$) and independent samples t tests were used for the comparative analyses between patients with prominent FNE and those with absent/mild FNE. Cramer's V for χ^2 tests and Cohen d for t-tests were computed as effect sizes for the significant results obtained in the comparative analyses and were interpreted as small (0.2-0.3), medium (0.4-0.7) and large (≥ 0.8). Also, variables where significant differences emerged in the comparative analyses were included in a multivariate logistic regression model with the backward conditional method to determine which variables (demographic and clinical) including the three main areas of internalized stigma are risk factors for prominent FNE in patients with schizophrenia. The alpha value for all tests was stablished at $p \leq 0.05$.

RESULTS

Sample Description

From the 269 patients included, 68.4% (n = 184) were men with a mean age of 37 years (S.D. = 10.7, range 18-68 years) and 11.6 years of education (S.D. = 3.1, range 2-21 years). Most of the patients were unemployed (72.1, n = 194) and single (98.9%, n = 266) at the time of the study. Age of illness onset was reported at age of 24 (S.D. = 7.8, range 9-51 years) with a mean duration of untreated psychosis (DUP) of 81.7 weeks (S.D. = 150.8, range 1-1776 weeks), approximately year and a half with overt psychotic symptoms without receiving specialized treatment for them. More than half of the patients had a history of a previous psychiatric hospitalization during illness course (56.1%, n = 151), with a mean number of 1.8 hospitalizations (S.D. = 1.7, range 1-15 hospitalizations).

Symptom severity at the time of the study according to the PANSS scale were as follows: positive subscale 15.8 mean score (S.D. = 5.6, range 8-38), negative subscale 16.9 mean score (S.D. = 4.9, range 7-35), cognitive subscale 14.5 mean score (S.D. = 3.9, range 4-29), excitability subscale 6.0 mean score (S.D. = 2.4, range 4-14), depression/anxiety subscale 7.1 mean score (S.D. = 2.7, range 4-16) and a total PANSS score of 60.4 (S.D. = 16.2, range 30-119).

The King's Internalized Stigma Scale (ISS) total score was 51.9 (S.D. = 15.3, range 6-84) with the following scores in the three scale dimensions: discrimination 23.4 (S.D. = 9.1, range 0-43), disclosure 20.0 (S.D. = 7.8, range 0-39) and positive aspects of mental illness 8.4 (S.D. = 3.3, 0-19). The total score of the BFNE-II scale was 19.9 (S.D. = 10.9, range 1-48). Using the upper quartile (75%) of the BFNE-II total score (27 points of the total score) to divide the sample, a total of 26.4% (n = 71) of the patients were classified as having prominent FNE and the remaining 73.6% (n = 198) with absent/mild FNE.

Table 1. Demographic and clinical features between patients with prominent FNE and absent/mild FNE

	Absent/mild FNE (n = 198)		Prominent FNE (n = 71)		Statistic
	n	%	n	%	
Sex					
Men	133	67.2	51	71.8	$\chi^2 = 0.52$, df 1, p = 0.46
Women	65	32.8	20	28.2	
Marital Status					
Single	195	98.5	71	100	$\chi^2 = 1.08$, df 1, p = 0.29
Married	3	1.5	--	--	
Employment Status					
Unemployed	144	72.7	50	70.4	$\chi^2 = 0.13$, df 1, p = 0.71
Employed	54	27.3	21	29.6	
Previous Hospitalization					
No	77	38.9	41	57.7	$\chi^2 = 7.54$, df 1, p = 0.006
Yes	121	61.1	30	42.3	Cramer's V = 0.16
	Mean	SD	Mean	SD	
Age	37.6	10.8	36.1	10.7	t = 0.98, df 267, p = 0.32
Years of Education	11.6	3.2	11.6	2.8	t = -0.05, df 267, p = 0.95
Age of Illness Onset (years)	24.3	7.8	24.1	7.7	t = 0.19, df 267, p = 0.84
DUP (weeks)	87.9	167.8	64.5	86.1	t = 1.12, df 267, p = 0.26
Age at First Hospitalization	27.0	7.9	26.5	8.0	t = 0.28, df 149, p = 0.77
Total Hospitalizations	1.8	1.8	1.7	1.2	t = 0.31, df 149, p = 0.75
PANSS					
Positive	15.7	5.4	15.7	6.4	t = - 0.08, df 267, p = 0.93
Negative	16.8	4.7	17.2	5.7	t = - 0.54, df 267, p = 0.58
Cognitive	14.5	3.9	14.5	4.1	t = - 0.16, df 267, p = 0.87
Excitement	5.9	2.4	6.1	2.5	t = - 0.66, df 267, p = 0.50
Depression/Anxiety	7.1	2.6	7.3	3.0	t = - 0.76, df 267, p = 0.44
Total	60.1	15.4	60.9	19.3	t = - 0.53, df 267, p = 0.59
King's Internalized Stigma					
Discrimination	21.9	9.0	27.6	8.1	t = - 4.64, df 267, p < 0.001 Cohen's d = 1.17
Disclosure	19.2	7.6	22.1	7.91	t = - 2.69, df 267, p = 0.007 Cohen's d = 0.41
Positive aspects	8.0	3.1	9.6	3.4	t = - 3.68, df 267, p < 0.001 Cohen's d = 0.94
Total	49.2	14.9	59.4	13.8	t = - 5.01, df 267, p < 0.001 Cohen's d = 0.82

Demographic and Clinical Features between Patients with Prominent FNE and Absent/Mild FNE

All demographic features (sex, age, years of education, marital status and occupation) and almost all clinical features, including symptom severity at the time of the study were similar among groups (Table 1). The only significant difference between groups was found in previous psychiatric hospitalizations where more patients with prominent FNE had a history of hospitalizations (61.1%, n = 121) when compared to those with absent/mild FNE (42.3%, n = 30; Cramer's V = 0.16, p = 0.006).

Internalized stigma was more severe in patient with prominent FNE. As seen in Table 1, dimensions and total score were higher in these patients than in those with mild/absent FNE with medium to large size effects.

Predictors of Fear of Negative Evaluation in Patients with Schizophrenia

According to the results in the comparative analysis, the following variables were included in a multivariate logistic model to determine which ones predict the presence of prominent FNE in patients with schizophrenia: 1) previous psychiatric hospitalizations, 2) discrimination dimension score, 3) disclosure dimension score and 3) positive aspects of mental illness dimension score. The final logistic regression model included the discrimination and the positive aspects dimensions of the King's internalized stigma scale as the most important predictors for prominent fear of negative evaluation in patients with schizophrenia (Table 2). The model can be considered as adequate according to the Hosmer & Lemeshaw goodness of fit value (p = 0.54).

Table 2. Logistic regression models for the prediction of prominent fear of negative evaluation in patients with schizophrenia

	β	OR	95% C.I.	p
Initial Model				
Previous hospitalization	-0.55	0.57	0.31 – 1.04	0.07
Discrimination	0.08	1.08	1.03 – 1.13	< 0.001
Disclosure	0.01	1.02	0.97 – 1.06	0.42
Positive aspects of mental illness	0.16	1.17	1.07 – 1.28	0.001
Final Model				
Discrimination	0.08	1.09	1.05 – 1.13	< 0.001
Positive aspects of mental illness	0.17	1.19	1.08 – 1.30	< 0.001

DISCUSSION

The aim of the present study was to determine the role of internalized stigma in the presence and severity of fear of negative evaluation in patients with schizophrenia.

Diagnosis and clinical follow-up of patients with this disorder is frequently centered in the assessment of the presence and severity of psychotic symptoms, primarily positive and negative symptoms. This may lead to the inappropriate assumption that all signs and symptoms experienced are reduced to the diagnostic criteria for schizophrenia (Kiran & Chaudhury, 2018). Important progress has been made as the impact of clinical comorbidities, such as affective and anxiety disorders, has been continuously remarked in the scientific literature and current diagnostic classifications (American Psychiatric Association, 2013; Gureje, 2018). However, in the daily clinical practice, some remnants of diagnostic reductionism may persist leading to a limited assessment of comorbid conditions in schizophrenia.

Social functioning refers to a state where an individual can effectively participate in social activities and understand others' social activities (Hiser & Koenigs, 2018). Impairment in social roles or social functioning has been a core feature of schizophrenia, found in first-episode patients as well as in chronic multi-episodes patients. Social evaluations are an integral part of social interactions and pronounced or extreme fears towards them may reflect a comorbid condition in these patients, namely social anxiety.

Although in the present study we did not determine a definite comorbid social anxiety disorder, we hypothesize that prominent FNE will be associated with some negative patient's clinical background such as younger age of illness onset, prolonged duration of untreated psychosis (DUP) and a greater number of psychiatric hospitalizations. Our results showed that patients with absent/mild and prominent FNE were very similar, both with an illness onset in the earlier 20's, with prolonged DUP – more than a year to receive specialized treatment for overt psychotic symptomatology, had between one and three psychiatric hospitalizations during their illness course and report similar symptom severity at the time of the study. These results add information to what was previously reported in the literature, particularly in terms of symptom severity. We expected more severe negative symptoms and affective symptoms (depression/anxiety PANSS dimension) in those patients with prominent FNE as negative symptoms have been conceived to share some common elements with social anxiety, such as apathy and avolition (Blanchard, et al., 1998; Kinoshita, et al., 2011), and the depression/anxiety dimension score was expected to reflect the anxiety secondary to FNE. However, this lack of differences also reflects the need to perform specific evaluations of other comorbidities and not to rely only in the symptom assessment severity reported by the PANSS, independently if it is used as a 3-dimensional (positive, negative and general dimensions) or a 5-dimensional scale (positive, negative, cognitive, excitement, depression/anxiety dimensions).

However, we found that fewer patients with prominent FNE had been hospitalized. These patients may be actively avoiding situations of social interaction leading to greater isolation and making clinical contact less probable. It is also likely that taking the patient to medical evaluation becomes even harder for the family, as the patient must be convinced not only of the benefits of medical evaluation but also that will not be negatively judged. This hypothesis should be taken with caution due to the size effect found in the statistical analysis and that the history of a psychiatric hospitalization was not a significant predictor for prominent FNE in patients with schizophrenia. However, future studies should direct efforts to assess features of social anxiety, if possible, since early stages of the disease.

Internalized stigma has a deleterious effect in persons with schizophrenia including poor quality of life, lower self-esteem, higher levels of anxiety, shame and isolation (Switaj, et al., 2009; Chuang, et al., 2019). In our study, prominent FNE was mainly explained by two important domains of internalized stigma named *discrimination* and *positive aspects of mental illness*. The first one, discrimination, refers to the perception of negative reaction of other people toward the illness, while higher scores on the positive aspects of the mental illness dimension refers to the lack of understanding and acceptance of illness (King, et al., 2007). We can either infer that FNE is not a causal phenomenon but a consequence of these aspects of internalized stigma or, on the other hand, prominent FNE could be a maintaining factor for internalized stigma. It is possible to conceive that patients with greater anxiety have a greater predisposition to prominent FNE in the context of external negative perceptions of the disease and may be at greater risk for internalizing stigma (Firmin, et al., 2017), leading to a continuous cycle of receiving, internalizing and living these negative experiences as anxiety and fear. In either case, our findings reflect the need to direct efforts for the design and implementation of specific interventions that effectively facilitate resisting stigma. Also, clinicians should carefully assess if social anxiety is present as a comorbid condition of schizophrenia and if so, assess its severity and interference with the patient's functionality and determine, if necessary, the most appropriate pharmacological management along with the needed therapeutic intervention, which may encompass internalized stigma and the management of fears of negative evaluation.

Despite the study limitations related to the cross-sectional nature of the study and the lack of a precise diagnosis of social anxiety, our study has two important implications for the treatment of patients with schizophrenia. First, the importance of performing an evaluation of other conditions that could affect patients with schizophrenia in order to provide effective treatment: anxiety symptoms generated by the fear of negative evaluation and the symptoms of schizophrenia; and second, the need to include internalized stigma as a treatment target for every patient due to its impact in prognosis, rehabilitation and daily living of patients.

REFERENCES

Aikawa, S., Kobayashi, H., Nemoto, T., Matsuo, S., Wada, Y., Mamiya, N., Yamaguchi, T., Katagiri, N., Tsujino, N. & Mizuno, M. (2018). Social anxiety and risk factors in patients with schizophrenia: Relationship with duration of untreated psychosis. *Psychiatry Research*, *263*, 94-100.

American Psychiatric Association (Ed.). (2013). Diagnostic and Statistical Manual of Mental Disorders 5th edition., DSM 5. Arlington, VA: American Psychiatric Association.

Blanchard, J. J., Mueser, K. T. & Bellack, A. S. (1998). Anhedonia, positive and negative affect, and social functioning in schizophrenia. *Schizophrenia Bulletin*, *24*, 413-424.

Bosanac, P., Mancuso, S. G. & Castle, D. J. (2016). Anxiety symptoms in psychotic disorders: results from the Second Australian National Mental Health Survey. *Clinical Schizophrenia and Related Psychoses*, *10*, 93-100.

Braga, R. J., Mendlowicz, M. V., Marrocos, R. P. & Figueira, I. L. (2005). Anxiety disorders in outpatients with schizophrenia: prevalence and impact on the subjective quality of life. *Journal of Psychiatric Research*, *39*, 409-414.

Carleton, R., Collimore, K. & Asmundson, G. (2007). Social anxiety and fear of negative evaluation: construct validity of the BFNE-II. *Journal of Anxiety Disorders*, *21*, 131-141.

Carleton, R., McCreary, D., Norton, P. & Asmundson, G. (2006). Brief fear of negative evaluation scale-revised. *Depression and Anxiety*, *23*, 297-303.

Chuang, S. P., Wu, J. Y. W. & Wang, C. S. (2019). Self-perception of mental illness and subjective and objective cognitive functioning in people with schizophrenia. *Neuropsychiatric Disease and Treatment*, *15*, 967-976.

Firmin, R. L., Luther, L., Salyers, M. P., Buck, K. D. & Lysaker, P. H. (2017). Greater metacognition and lower fear of negative evaluation: Potential factors contributing to improved stigma resistance among individuals diagnosed with schizophrenia. *Israel Journal of Psychiatry and Related Sciences*, *54*, 50-54.

First, M. B., Spitzer, R. L., Williams, J. B. & Gibbon, M. (1997). Structured Clinical Interview for DSM-IV Disorders (SCID). *American Psychiatric Association*, Washington, DC.

Flores-Reynoso, S., Medina, R. & Robles, R. (2011). Study of the Spanish translation and psychometric assessment of a scale to measure internalized stigma in patients with severe mental disorders. *Salud Mental*, *24*, 333-339.

Fresán, A., De la Fuente-Sandoval, C., Loyzaga, C., García-Anaya, M., Meyenberg, N., Nicolini, H. & Apiquian, R. (2005). A forced five-dimensional factor analysis and concurrent validity of the positive and negative syndrome scale (PANSS) in Mexican schizophrenic patients. *Schizophrenia Research*, *72*, 123-129.

Fresán, A. & Robles-García, R. (2011). Illness recognition and beliefs about treatment for schizophrenia in a community sample of Mexico City: Differences according to personality traits. In: Melissa E. Jordan. *Personality Traits: Theory, Testing and Influence*. Nova Science Publishers, Inc., pp. 145-154. ISBN: 978-1-61728-934-7.

Gullone, E. (2000). The development of normal fear: a century of research. *Clinical Psychologial Review*, *20*, 429-451.

Gureje, O. (2018). ICD-11 chapter on mental and behavioural disorders: heralding new ways of seeing old problems. *Epidemiology and Psychiatric Sciences*, *27*, 209-211.

Hiser, J. & Koenigs, M. (2018). The multifaceted role of the ventromedial prefrontal cortex in emotion, decision making, social cognition, and psychopathology. *Biological Psychiatry*, *83*, 638-647.

Kay, S., Fiszbein, A., Opler, Vital-Herne M. & Fuentes, L. S. (1990). The Positive and Negative Syndrome Scale-Spanish adaptation. *Journal of Nervous and Mental Disease*, *178*, 510-517.

King, M., Dinos, S., Shaw, J., Watson, R., Stevens, S., Passetti, F., Weich, S. & Serfaty, M. (2007). The stigma scale: development of a standardized measure of the stigma of mental illness. *British Journal of Psychiatry*, *190*, 248-254.

Kinoshita, Y., Kingdon, D., Kinoshita, K., Kinoshita, Y., Saka, K., Arisue, Y., Dayson, D., Nakaaki, S., Fukuda, K., Yoshida, K., Harris, S. & Furukawa, T. A. (2011). Fear of negative evaluation is associated with delusional ideation in non-clinical population and patients with schizophrenia. *Social Psychiatry and Psychiatric Epidemiology*, *46*, 703-710.

Kiran, C. & Chaudhury, S. (2018). Correlates and management of comorbid anxiety disorders in schizophrenia. *Industrial Psychiatry Journal*, *27*, 271-278.

Leary, M. (1983). A brief version of the Fear of Negative Evaluation Scale. *Personality and Social Psychology Bulletin*, *9*, 371-375.

Lysaker, P. H., Yanos, P. T., Outcalt, J. & Roe, D. (2010). Association of stigma, self-esteem, and symptoms with concurrent and prospective assessment of social anxiety in schizophrenia. *Clinical Schizophrenia and Related Psychoses*, *4*, 41–48.

McEnery, C., Lim, M. H., Tremain, H., Knowles, A. & Alvarez-Jimenez, M. (2019). Prevalence rate of social anxiety disorder in individuals with a psychotic disorder: A systematic review and meta-analysis. *Schizophrenia Research*, *208*, 25-33.

Michail, M. & Birchwood, M. (2014). Social anxiety in first-episode psychosis: the role of childhood trauma and adult attachment. *Journal of Affective Disorders*, *163*, 102–109.

Michail, M., Birchwood, M. & Tait, L. (2017). Systematic review of cognitive-behavioural therapy for social anxiety disorder in psychosis. *Brain Sciences*, *7*, 45.

Mobbs, D. (2018). The ethological deconstruction of fear(s). *Current Opinion in Behavioral Sciences*, *24*, 32-37.

Pallanti, S., Quercioli, L. & Hollander, E. (2004). Social anxiety in outpatients with schizophrenia: a relevant cause of disability. *American Journal of Psychiatry*, *161*, 53–58.

Rector, N., Kocovski, N. & Ryder, A. (2006). Social anxiety and the fear of causing discomfort to others. *Cognitive Therapy and Research*, *30*, 279-296.

Reichenberger, J., Smyth, J. M. & Blechert, J. (2018). Fear of evaluation unpacked: day-to-day correlates of fear of negative and positive evaluation. *Anxiety, Stress and Coping*, *31*, 159-174.

Robles-García, R., Páez, F., Fresán, A., Tejero, J., Lomelí, M. & Padilla, C. (2012). Is it me? Fears of causing discomfort to others and of negative evaluation as predictors of social anxiety in men and women form a community sample of Mexico. In: Anna S. Morales. *Trait Anxiety*. Nova Publishers, Inc. p.p. 155-169. ISBN: 978-1-61324-551-4.

Switaj, P., Wciórka, J., Smolarska-Switaj, J. & Grygiel, P. (2009). Extent and predictors of stigma experienced by patients with schizophrenia. *European Psychiatry*, *24*, 513–520.

INDEX

A

abnormalities, 12, 16, 31, 33, 35, 71, 72, 99
access, 37, 55, 59, 76
ADHD, 27, 29, 36, 63, 69, 70
adolescents, 63, 69
adults, 18, 36, 42, 49, 60, 71
affective disorder, 9, 65, 120
age, 1, 11, 17, 18, 19, 25, 29, 36, 37, 60, 77, 93, 106, 107, 109, 112, 114, 116
aggression, 32, 43, 109
American Psychiatric Association, 108, 115, 118, 119
antipsychotic, 67, 78, 79, 85, 91, 92, 110
anti-psychotic, 41
antipsychotic drugs, 67, 78, 79
anxiety, 14, 29, 49, 53, 55, 57, 59, 64, 70, 95, 106, 107, 108, 109, 111, 112, 113, 115, 116, 117, 118, 120, 121
anxiety disorder, 70, 115, 120
assessment, 2, 4, 10, 11, 13, 21, 28, 42, 63, 66, 77, 107, 110, 111, 115, 116, 119, 120
attitudes, 3, 106, 109
auditory perception, 8
autism, 26, 64
avoidance, 31, 106, 108
awareness, 3, 19, 28, 32, 36, 40

B

behavior therapy, 65, 70
behavioral neuropsychology, 4
behaviors, 2, 4, 5, 14, 32, 39, 43, 52, 53, 54, 63, 109
benefits, 14, 40, 52, 56, 77, 116
biomarkers, 75, 76, 77, 79, 82, 83, 85, 86, 87, 88, 90, 91, 92, 93, 96, 98, 99, 100, 101, 102
bipolar disorder, 49, 61, 62, 67, 69
blood, 75, 76, 77, 78, 79, 80, 81, 82, 83, 86, 87, 88, 89, 90, 91, 92, 93, 94, 95, 96, 97, 99, 100, 101, 102, 103, 104
brain, 2, 3, 4, 5, 8, 9, 10, 11, 12, 16, 21, 22, 24, 28, 29, 31, 32, 33, 34, 36, 38, 62, 63, 65, 69, 71, 76, 80, 84, 87, 88, 89, 93
brain activity, 3, 28
brain damage, 11, 28, 33, 36
brain structure, 2, 12

C

candidates, 77, 82, 84, 86
caregivers, 35, 37
cell cycle, 85, 86
cell death, 31, 82

central nervous system, 4, 77, 82, 89
childhood, 28, 47, 48, 53, 72, 108, 120
children, 11, 14, 17, 18, 28, 29, 64, 66, 70, 71
classification, 8, 23, 24, 37, 102, 115
classification disorder, 8
clinical neuropsychology, 4, 64, 65
clinical psychology, 1, 4
coding, 84, 89
cognition, 4, 5, 61, 63, 82, 83
cognitive abilities, 10, 11, 28, 37, 44
cognitive deficit, 2, 24, 34
cognitive deficits, 2, 24, 34
cognitive flexibility, 33, 34, 71
cognitive function, 4, 5, 9, 10, 34, 35, 44, 64, 69, 119
cognitive neuropsychology, 4, 62, 64
cognitive performance, 5, 10, 13
cognitive process, 22, 106, 109
cognitive processing, 22, 106, 109
cognitive rehabilitation, 39, 59, 61, 66
cognitive skills, 10, 38, 59, 60
cognitive-behavioral therapy, 36, 55, 56, 57, 58, 59, 62
communication, 2, 12, 39, 44, 49, 50, 63
communication skills, 39, 63
communication skills and socializing, 39
community, 37, 42, 51, 55, 59, 60, 67, 119, 121
complexity, 33, 72, 75, 93
compliance, 55, 72
complications, 31, 37
computer, 25, 26, 38, 56
construct validity, 111, 118
continuous performance test, 27, 63
control group, 25, 83, 93
coordination, 39, 45
correlation, 3, 81, 92, 93
cortex, 10, 12, 23, 30, 31, 34, 64, 70
creativity, 32, 34
criticism, 46, 106, 109
cytokines, 77, 80, 81

D

defects, 9, 28, 29, 31
deficiencies, 10, 11, 37
deficiency, 28, 32
delusions, 6, 12, 30
dementia, 26, 29, 71
depression, 28, 29, 48, 49, 55, 56, 60, 65, 111, 112, 116
detection, 25, 66, 93
Diagnostic and Statistical Manual of Mental Disorders, 69, 118
diagnostic criteria, 2, 34, 115
disability, 29, 30, 121
disclosure, 107, 111, 112, 114
discomfort, 108, 121
discrimination, 69, 106, 107, 109, 111, 112, 114, 117
diseases, 29, 37, 39, 47, 48, 60, 89
disorder, 1, 7, 25, 29, 31, 32, 33, 34, 35, 40, 41, 56, 58, 65, 67, 89, 106, 107, 108, 109, 115, 116, 120
distress, 11, 108
diversity, 52, 66
DNA, 85, 94, 98
dopamine, 32, 40, 65, 71, 78, 79
dopaminergic, 32, 78
drug therapy, 31, 36, 39, 51, 60
drug treatment, 31, 78, 79
drugs, 37, 40, 41, 67
DSM-IV-TR, 106, 110

E

eating disorders, 48, 63, 71
education, 1, 39, 47, 49, 50, 112, 114
emotion, 46, 64, 119
emotional problems, 29, 52
endophenotypes, 77, 82
energy, 12, 87

environment, 12, 14, 29, 32, 34, 36, 43, 44, 52, 53, 56
equipment, 42, 44, 47
etiology, 30, 75, 77, 80, 83, 86, 91
everyday life, 9, 56
evidence, 33, 48, 50, 51, 55, 59, 71, 90
executive function, 25, 27, 32, 33, 35, 36, 62, 64, 66, 70, 72
executive functioning, 27, 35, 64, 66
executive functions, 32, 33, 35, 36, 70
exercise, 36, 62
experimental neuropsychology, 4, 63
exposure, 31, 59

F

families, 29, 39, 47
family members, 2, 28, 42, 48, 49, 50, 51, 58
family relationships, 48, 49
family therapy, 39, 47, 48, 49, 50, 51, 63, 64, 70
fear, 9, 54, 106, 107, 108, 109, 111, 114, 115, 117, 118, 119, 120, 121
fear of negative evaluation, 106, 107, 108, 109, 111, 114, 115, 118, 119, 120
fears, 59, 115, 117
feelings, 30, 46, 55, 56, 57, 58, 59
fitness, 21, 32
flexibility, 9, 24, 34, 47
fMRI, 34, 62
formation, 24, 89
frontal, 6, 7, 9, 12, 23, 25, 26, 28, 31, 32, 33, 38, 62
frontal cortex, 10, 12, 23, 31
frontal lobe, 9, 25, 26, 32

G

gene expression, 76, 77, 79, 80, 81, 82, 86, 88, 89, 91, 93, 95, 96, 97, 99, 101, 102, 103, 104
genes, 2, 32, 75, 76, 77, 80, 82, 84, 85, 87, 88, 89, 90
genetic factors, 31, 32
genetics, 75, 97, 98, 99, 102
genome, 82, 86, 90
glia, 31, 81
gray matter, 31, 33, 68
group therapy, 35, 39, 51, 52, 53, 54, 55
growth, 31, 80, 84, 91
growth factor, 31, 80

H

hallucinations, 12, 30
health, 27, 37, 39, 42, 60, 69
hearing impairment, 8
hemisphere, 6, 12, 28, 29, 65
heterogeneity, 65, 76
hippocampus, 30, 31, 33
histone, 84, 89
history, 11, 64, 107, 108, 110, 112, 114, 116
hopelessness, 106, 109
hospitalization, 28, 37, 38, 39, 40, 47, 60, 64, 93, 112, 115, 117
hospitalizations, viii, xi, 2, 28, 37, 38, 39, 40, 47, 60, 64, 93, 107, 110, 112, 113, 114, 115, 116, 117
hostility, 44, 46, 50
human, 2, 7, 77, 108
hyperactivity, 25, 26, 27, 49
hypothesis, 31, 32, 35, 65, 71, 79, 80, 116

I

identification, 76, 77, 93

images, 15, 45
immune system, 32, 80, 82, 83
inattention, 27, 49
independence, 42, 43, 44
individuals, 1, 3, 5, 10, 11, 26, 31, 32, 35, 36, 48, 53, 76, 90, 106, 108, 109, 119, 120
inhibition, 7, 22, 32, 33, 34, 35, 63
initiation, 82, 86
injuries, 5, 9, 11, 26, 32
injury, 2, 3, 4, 6, 7, 8, 10, 11, 21, 24, 28, 33, 42
intelligence, 10, 13, 14, 15, 16, 17, 18, 61, 66, 67, 68, 70, 71, 72
internalization, x, xi, 106, 107, 109
internalized stigma, v, vii, x, xi, 105, 106, 107, 109, 111, 112, 113, 114, 115, 117, 118, 119
interpersonal relations, 34, 43
interpersonal relationships, 34, 43
intervention, 55, 85, 117
isolation, 37, 50, 51, 109, 116, 117
issues, 9, 19, 37

J

Jordan, 64, 119

L

lead, 8, 15, 31, 37, 42, 59, 108, 115
learning, 3, 10, 19, 23, 28, 29, 34, 42, 54, 63, 73
learning disabilities, 28, 29, 63, 73
left hemisphere, 6, 12, 16, 28, 65
leisure, 29, 42
lesions, 25, 34
loci, 88, 90
locus, 90, 91

M

magnetic resonance, 33, 34, 72
magnetic resonance imaging, 33, 34
malingering, 66, 67
management, 45, 59, 117, 120
MBP, 80, 85, 101
measurement, 5, 11, 14
medical, 1, 40, 51, 57, 78, 110, 116
medication, 31, 38, 40, 42, 50, 51, 55, 62, 65, 67, 72, 78, 80, 94, 99, 103
memory, 7, 8, 9, 10, 11, 19, 23, 29, 33, 37, 67, 69
memory impairment, 9
mental activity, 2, 9
mental disorder, 2, 5, 11, 27, 28, 30, 33, 44, 56, 60, 61, 75, 106, 108, 109, 119
mental health, 38, 39, 47, 52, 56, 59
mental illness, 33, 47, 48, 52, 55, 57, 93, 107, 111, 112, 114, 115, 117, 119, 120
messages, 7, 8
meta-analysis, 36, 63, 67, 69, 70, 92, 120
metabolism, 77, 87
Mexico, 68, 105, 110, 119, 121
miRNA, 76, 89, 90, 91
misunderstanding, 2, 58
models, 5, 49, 64
mood disorder, 48, 49, 85
motivation, 5, 31
motor dysfunction, 7
motor skills, 29, 32
MRI, 65, 68, 70
mRNA, 78, 79, 80, 81, 83, 84, 85, 86, 87, 88, 90
mRNAs, 81, 82
mutations, 76, 85

N

National Academy of Sciences, 98, 102
nerve, 31, 85

Index

neurons, 31, 81
neuropsychological function, 1, 2, 6, 27, 30, 31, 35, 36, 64, 68, 70
neuropsychological tests, 5, 10, 13, 21
neuropsychology, 1, 3, 4, 5, 28, 35, 62, 63, 64, 65, 68, 69, 71
neuroscience, 2, 3, 4, 5, 10, 13, 28, 29, 32, 37
neurotransmitter, 40, 79
neurotransmitters, 40, 77, 78, 79
nutrition, 28, 60

O

occipital, 7, 68, 72
occupational therapy, 39, 42, 43, 44, 62, 66, 68
organ, 38, 87
organize, 8, 15
outpatient, 38, 55, 108, 110
outpatients, 118, 121

P

parents, 29, 49
parietal, 6, 7, 34, 72, 73
participants, 20, 21, 22, 39, 52, 54
pathophysiology, 80, 91
pathway, 12, 65, 82, 86, 87
pathways, 29, 76, 77, 84, 86
peripheral blood, 76, 77, 81, 87, 90, 91, 92
peripheral blood mononuclear cell, 91, 92
personal health education, 39
personality, 8, 9, 15, 53, 119
personality disorder, 9, 53, 97
personality traits, 9, 15, 119
phenotype, 83, 85, 86, 90, 93
phenotypes, 76, 77, 83, 86
physiology, 6, 31
population, 30, 68, 76, 84, 88, 93, 111
prefrontal cortex, 34, 119

principles, 4, 5, 17, 23, 48, 53, 55, 56, 64
problem-solving, 10, 26, 32, 36
professional rehabilitation, 60
professional skills, 39
prognosis, 77, 79, 92, 118
proteins, 80, 84, 85
psychiatric disorder, 1, 80, 87, 89
psychiatric disorders, 80, 87, 89
psychiatric patients, 30, 37, 55
psychiatrist, 40, 110
psychologist, 11, 17, 40, 55, 57
psychology, 2, 3, 4, 5, 70
psychopathology, 5, 81, 119
psychoses, 4, 68
psychosis, 59, 61, 62, 71, 79, 80, 87, 110, 112, 116, 118, 120
psychotherapy, 40, 52, 55, 67
psychotic symptomatology, 107, 116
psychotic symptoms, 112, 115

Q

quality of life, 37, 50, 106, 108, 117, 118
quartile, 107, 111, 112
quetiapine, 67, 78

R

reaction time, 64, 72
reading, 28, 29
reality, 46, 51, 58, 75
reasoning, 10, 23, 30, 32
recall, 9, 11
receptor, 78, 79, 80, 81, 84, 88
receptors, 32, 78, 81, 82, 83
recognition, 64, 119
recovery, 40, 106, 109
regression, 85, 90, 107, 111, 114, 115
regression analysis, 85, 90, 107
regression model, 111, 114, 115

rehabilitation, 35, 36, 37, 38, 39, 42, 47, 52, 59, 61, 62, 66, 67, 72, 118
relatives, 64, 89
reliability, 14, 15, 24
remission, 86, 88
replication, 83, 85
researchers, 2, 6, 12, 25, 33, 36, 76
resources, 39, 60
response, 14, 22, 23, 30, 31, 33, 34, 63, 77, 79, 83, 88, 91, 92, 106, 109
right hemisphere, 6, 16, 28, 29
risk, 31, 63, 64, 67, 69, 72, 77, 89, 90, 93, 107, 112, 117, 118
risk assessment, 31, 77
risk factors, 31, 63, 67, 107, 112, 118
risperidone, 78, 92
RNA, 84, 87, 90, 94, 98
RNAs, 84, 89, 99

S

schizophrenia, 6, 11, 12, 13, 25, 26, 30, 31, 32, 33, 34, 35, 37, 38, 39, 40, 42, 44, 47, 48, 49, 50, 51, 52, 53, 55, 56, 57, 58, 59, 60, 61, 62, 63, 64, 65, 66, 67, 68, 69, 70, 71, 72, 73, 75, 76, 77, 78, 79, 80, 81, 82, 83, 84, 85,86, 87, 88, 89, 90, 91, 92, 93, 94, 95, 96, 97, 99, 100, 101, 102, 103, 104, 105, 106, 107, 108, 109, 110, 112, 114, 115, 117, 118, 119, 120, 121
schizophrenic patients, 35, 37, 42, 44, 56, 62, 78, 80, 81, 86, 89, 119
science, 2, 3, 69
second generation, 41, 70
selective attention, 22, 23, 27
self-esteem, 14, 42, 46, 53, 106, 109, 117, 120
sensitivity, 61, 89, 93, 109
serotonin, 71, 78
services, 37, 38, 42, 47, 51, 60, 62, 68, 108, 110
sex, 64, 84, 114
shape, 7, 22, 24
shock, 39, 60
showing, 32, 76
side effects, 40, 41, 51, 55, 70
signaling pathway, 83, 84
signs, 8, 40, 64, 93, 115
simple reaction time, 22, 64, 72
skills training, 42, 65
social anxiety, 106, 107, 108, 116, 117, 120, 121
social cognition, 34, 62, 119
social interaction, 46, 106, 108, 115, 116
social interactions, 106, 108, 115
social situations, 42, 106
social skills, 14, 38, 39, 60, 68
social workers, 42, 59
society, 37, 38
spatial memory, 7
spatial orientation, 7
specialists, 47, 52, 68
speech, 6, 28, 43, 55, 56
standard deviation, 19, 111
Stanford-Binet test, 17, 18
state, 12, 14, 26, 86, 89, 91, 93, 115
stigma, 106, 107, 109, 111, 112, 114, 115, 117, 118, 119, 120, 121
stigmatized, 106, 109
stimulus, 12, 22, 23
stress, 31, 54, 57, 58, 59, 82
stretching exercises, 38
structure, 3, 49, 71, 72, 89, 91
Sun, 62, 92, 100, 102
survival, 82, 106, 108
susceptibility, 32, 76, 88
symptoms, 2, 6, 12, 27, 28, 30, 33, 35, 38, 40, 42, 44, 47, 49, 50, 55, 57, 58, 59, 60, 61, 64, 67, 76, 77, 78, 79, 82, 93, 106, 107, 108, 109, 110, 111, 115, 116, 118, 120
syndrome, 30, 71, 73, 90, 119

T

T cell, 78, 80
T cells, 78, 80
target, 26, 90, 91, 118
team members, 54, 59
techniques, 11, 39, 50, 56, 93
temporal, 6, 7, 8, 9, 18, 33, 62, 64, 69, 97
temporal lobe, 7, 8, 9, 69
testing, 11, 18, 51, 71
therapeutic work, 42, 65
therapist, 42, 44, 51, 54, 55, 57, 58
therapy, 35, 39, 42, 43, 44, 47, 48, 49, 50, 51, 52, 53, 54, 55, 56, 57, 58, 59, 61, 62, 63, 64, 65, 68, 70, 72, 120
thoughts, 30, 32, 56, 57, 58
tissue, 32, 33, 35, 76, 77, 88, 90
TNF, 80, 81, 85, 94, 97
Tower of London Test, 25
Trail Making Test, 21, 63, 66
training, 39, 42
traits, 32, 93
transcription, 77, 82, 84, 91
transcription factors, 82, 84, 91
translation, 77, 82, 119
trauma, 26, 120
treatment, 10, 28, 36, 37, 38, 39, 40, 41, 42, 44, 47, 48, 49, 50, 51, 52, 53, 54, 55, 56, 57, 58, 59, 60, 62, 63, 65, 67, 70, 71, 72, 77, 78, 79, 86, 88, 89, 91, 92, 106, 107, 109, 110, 112, 116, 117, 119
trial, 63, 67
twins, 32, 69

V

variables, 14, 106, 109, 111, 114
verbal fluency, 20, 62, 69
verbal fluency test, 20, 62
vision, 6, 57, 68
visual perception disorder, 8
visual-spatial diagnosis, 7

W

Wechsler Adult Intelligence Scale, 13, 66
Wechsler Intelligence Scale, 11, 13, 14, 15, 16, 67, 72
Wechsler Memory Test, 19
Wisconsin, 9, 12, 23, 24, 65, 70, 71
Wisconsin Card Matching Task, 23
working memory, 35, 70
worldwide, 76, 106, 109